MANAGE AL.

NECK PAIN

CERVICAL SPONDYLOSIS

READ INSIDE

Cure And Manipulate Neck Pain
Learn Accurate Neck Exercises
Use Simple Homoeopathic Remedies
Eat Befitting Diet To Fight The Disease
Avoid Disease By Change Of Life Style
Cure By Alternative Therapies And Yoga
Basic Questions Relating To Neck Pain

Dr. Shiv Dua

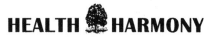

HEALTH 🌳 HARMONY

An imprint of

B. Jain Publishers (P) Ltd.

MANAGE AND CURE NECK PAIN CERVICAL SPONDYLOSIS

First Edition: 2003
4th Impression: 2013

> **NOTE FROM THE PUBLISHERS**
> Any information given in this book is not intended to be taken as a replacement for medical advice. Any person with a condition requiring medical attention should consult a qualified practitioner or therapist.

Published by Kuldeep Jain for

HEALTH 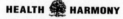 **HARMONY**

An Imprint of

B. JAIN PUBLISHERS (P) LTD.
1921/10, Chuna Mandi, Paharganj, New Delhi 110 055 (INDIA)
Tel.: +91-11-4567 1000   Fax: +91-11-4567 1010
Email: info@bjain.com   Website: **www.bjain.com**

Printed in India by
JJ Imprints Pvt. Ltd.

ISBN: 978-81-319-0192-2

DEDICATION

THIS BOOK is dedicated to **Geological Survey of India (GSI)** and my retrospect, the jungle and camp life in Drilling Division of this department.

GSI gave me spate of time in serene solitude of my tents to realize actual meaning of life and meditate over social-latitude away from restrictions of social rituals in the society. GSI widened my area of thinking and fetched me academic achievements. It is again GSI, which anchored me to euphoria of literary-guzzle and many of my field-life stories got published in English and Hindi magazines. Even after retirement from service, it is the inspiration and attitudes developed in solitary life of GSI, which enabled me to write four books on Homoeopathy within a span of five years. GSI induced in me a sense of total satisfaction although it did not gave me a single promotion in my cadre.

When I entered the solitary jungle life of tents, I was only a matriculate. I did my master of arts (M.A.) in English, Honors in Hindi (Parbhakar), Diploma and Degree in Homoeopathy (D.I.Hom. and H.M.D., both from British Institute of Homoeopathy, London) through correspondence, while working as a Driller. My transfers from states to states like Rajasthan, Bihar, Orissa, West Bengal, Manipur, Assam, Madhya Pradesh, and Maharashtra and in countries like Bhutan reverberated me chances to probe inscrutable jungles and know innocent villagers. Although this type of sojourn filled me up with nostalgia being away from family life yet I managed to conceive it as a parable of service to people. I diverted my time to treat and cure poor villagers, who lived in remote jungles away from facilities of medical-femininities. My kit of homoeopathic medicines always traveled with me in the tents, pitched in jungles, hills and deserts. It is paradoxical that a highly responsible gazette post of driller could snatch time from its routine to deviate to exuberant and jaunty therapy like Homoeopathy.

I feel it my duty to thank the **Director General and all officers of GSI,** a department where I served for 37 years. The officers and the staff encouraged me, helped me and remained with me even during the difficult times when I was their representative (General Secretary of Drilling Officers Association). I like to pay regards to Late shri C. Cheriyan, Ex-Director (Drilling) who was like a teacher to me in my professional and personal etiquettes. His guidance and inspiration remains with me even now.

I am also thankful to my colleagues and friends namely K.P.Duttaburman, R.Krishnan, C.P.Dusad, R.K.Khanna, C.L.Rajendra Kumar, R.L.Gera, N.S.Sodha, Ghansham Lal, S.C.Samanta, Bhopal Datta, Rajinder Singh, O.P.Sharma and H.S.Virk besides all the staff associated with my unit-works in GSI from time to time.

Dr. Shiv Dua

A WORD OF THANKS

I am thankful to **Dr. P.N.Jain** for his dynamic contribution to the cause of homoeopathy through pioneering this great publication house, **M/s B.Jain Publishers.** It is his constituent and continuous tireless effort that this firm is crowning Homoeopathy with a glory. Can anyone imagine the blossoming growth of modern Homoeopathic Medical Colleges and study-courses without garnishing the help of books published by **M/s B. Jain Publishers.**

I must mention the name of **Shri Kuldeep Jain** of M/s **B.Jain Publishers** whose gorgeous wisdom to suggest an appropriate subject for a book on cervical spondylosis inspired me to write this book. Shri Kuldeep possesses an institutional instinct with which he integrates the work of his authors. When I presented the manuscript of my last book on 'Thyroid', he examined it through a brief scanning within a minute and accepted it for publishing without referring it to his team of expert doctors. It is this logistic ability and reliance, which has earned him a noble name in the field of homoeopathic publications.

Dr. Shiv Dua

PREFACE

THERE IS a popular saying in America that death and taxes are unavoidable. So is the case with backache and neck pain. During one's lifetime, these pains are bound to occur, may be temporary but everyone experiences these pains in mild or acute form.

During a meeting with Shri Kuldeep Jain in his chamber, (M/s B.Jain Publishers), it was pointed out by Shri Kuldeep that there is a tremendous increase in the number of patients suffering from cervical spondylosis and there is an urgent necessity for a book to guide the sufferers. They mostly depend upon intake of modern medicines consisting of antibiotics and pain killing agents. Their prolonged use makes the pathogenic infection or bacteria resistant to the drugs besides that they produce side effects. They also interfere with the metabolic process of the body and may produce different diseases or allergic reactions. This was the subject in which I had worked hard and made several experiments during my practice of more than three decades and I decided to write on this most wanted subject of the day.

There was another primary reason why I liked the subject to be explored. You may not believe it but explanation here is essential. People belonging to North West Frontier Province of

Pakistan (NWFP) and especially hailing from Dera Ismail Khan know that "DUA" clans are blessed with certain healing powers and Dua's are supposed to be good doctors, so thought the people of D.I.Khan. It was in this belief that people suffering from neck pain and backache used to visit Dua's houses in the early morning, before sunrise, *to get a pat or pushing-touch. This act on the part of a Dua family used to cure the pains of the sufferers.*

When my father shifted to Amritsar in Punjab after partition of India, this tradition was kept alive because people there knew about these blessings imparted on Dua's. They used to throng our house not only for this but also for taking homoeopathic pills from my father who practiced Homoeopathy on charity. I was about eight years of age and I was ordered by my father to do the job of pushing on his behalf. I remember to have pushed or patted people suffering from neck pains or back pains hundreds of time. Along with the pushing act, I was told by my father to secretly recite 'Gayatri Mantra' and salute the name of my grandfather, who was a renowned Saint of his time. This worked well. Even today, those who believe in this aspect of blessings, come to our residence. I also advise them to take homoeopathic medicines from my chamber at Arya Samaj Hospital, Sector 19, Faridabad. Only faith does not cure.

So, the subject was fascinating to me and here is a book written on my experience and clues from literature. It will be of value if someone gets or inducts relief to patients after reading this book.

Dr. Shiv Dua

INTRODUCTION

WHEN WE think about the subject of this book, cervical spondylosis, we must remember that it is one of the innumerous diseases, a human body can have. Our body is an amazing living machine, which cannot be devised or manufactured by humans. In our majestic structure, it is the head, which contains the body's control and communication through our brains. The head may not be moving much but brains cannot remain silent in its activities. It goes on directing the torso, thorax, abdomen, hands and feet to prove that the body is living. All our systems have to cooperate under the control of brain. Brain, a pinkish gray organ with cheese like consistency weighing about three pounds, is such a wonderful tool in the body, which has not been fully probed about its exact functioning modes. Physiologically, it has the same structure in every one and still it works differently in each body, so far its output is concerned. With the same structure of brain, someone becomes a priest and the other a robber; some one is savior and the other a killer. What is it that makes such a difference? Is this trend inherent or cultivated or acquired from the environmental social set-up, which develops a tendency or an attitude? Is it due to the congenital effects developed in the brain? How is it that someone has tendency to commit suicide and the other is afraid of even a slight pinch on his skin? It is a dilemma still now when the medical science boasts of many achievements. How big is a brain, which makes a person change over-night. Well, it is about two percent of the total body weight and yet it consumes about twenty five percent of total energy, a body possesses. Such consumption of energy is through billions of nerve cells and trillions of nerve connections.

Why did I start from the brain in this introduction of the book? It is from here that our nervous system functions and makes link with the neck and spinal cord. It is the spine, collarbone, shoulder blade and rib cage, which concern our subject of cervical. Cervical means relating to the neck or a cervix and cervical spondylosis is inflammation of the cervical vertebras. Vertebra is the bony segment of the spinal column. Why should there be inflammation of the cervical vertebra? This is very important question but we do not have a rational looking answer to this. It is in the same way as stated above in the case of mysterious behavior of mind or brain. The modern upgraded knowledge of human body links this question with the modern style of living of people, especially urban. The people in big cities have a very fast life so far their working is concerned but they lead a sedentary style of living utilizing maximum of mechanical gadgets and minimum of body effort. They sit hours after hours before the computers and TV screens or conduct continuous type of studies, lowering the neck and making least of movements of neck for a longer time. These people do not believe in open-air exercises or have no time to spare for this.

During my spell of leading life in villages and jungles for more than three decades, while working in Geological Survey of India, I have seen very few cases of cervical spondylosis. These cases also had a background of city dwelling with abundant sedentary profession. Leaving aside the cases of accidents and traumas, I have not seen villagers wearing neck collars to straighten their necks. As a matter of fact, we, the 'educated' class people belonging to middle or higher groups of society, have not adopted the correct style of living. We are religiously following the use of latest electronic or mechanical gadgets denoting the advancement of science and technology but forgetting the old values of life where body exercise and physical work was of much importance.

I beg your pardon, if I am wrong, but it is a fact that cervical spondylosis is the invention of modern 'educated' lot, which believes in less of physical work and more of mental work. It is very common to see people working for more than 8 hours on the desk or before a computer or drive vehicles continuously for many hours. It is these people who will be found making complaint of the disease. It is not that all those who work in the above fashion suffer from spondylosis. It is those who ignore the rules of maintaining good health through physical exercise in a proper fashion. We have examples of towering personalities like Gandhi ji, Nehru, Lincoln, Churchill and many others who worked for more than 16 hours a day but never had this trouble. They had talented qualities of work associated with regular habit of physical exercise.

The tragedy of our life is that **we are unable to do a thing we know to be right.** We know physical exercise is essential but we do not follow this. Not only this, when we know that certain postures of body while studying, too much of stooping for longer time, too long sitting before the computer etc. are some of the reasons for this disease, **we are unable to desist from doing this wrong.** It is the human nature that we know we should lead a moral life and yet we commit sinful acts. We know habit of smoking leads to disastrous diseases and still we cling to it. We consult doctors in case of any problem as a consequence of this habit but would not leave the habit.

This book is written to benefit both common mass and the students of homoeopathy or even practitioners. I have tried my best to see that complicated medical terms are not used and if unavoidable to do so, the meaning of the term has been defined. It is not the anatomy or physiology of the neck glands or spine, the common man is interested in. The interest of the people is to know the remedial measures, the medicines, the exercises, the living style improvement, the diet changes and the right corrected suggestions of manipulative measures. All possible help has been taken from alternative therapies without any biased feeling for a single therapy because the objective is to benefit and absolute benefit to relieve the patient of this most common disease of the cities.

Dr. Shiv Dua
M.A., D.I.Hom., HMD
2617, Sector-16,
Faridabad-121 002
Phone: 0129-2281764
E-mail: shiv_dua@hotmail.com

HOMOEOPATHY & OSTEOPATHY

IN 1828, when Dr. S. Hahnemann, founder of Homoeopathy, wrote a book 'Chronic Diseases', it opened a new chapter in the world of medicine. Exactly during this year, another genius Dr. Andrew Tailer Still was born in US. Hahnemann had taken a different path to heal the community of ills, which was not very much liked by the doctors of the times. Dr. Still also made a history by opening a new theory to a world of obstinate traditional medicine. *Still founded a manipulative therapy called osteopathy.* This man had a rare vision and perseverance for doing something new. He was a strong and sturdy man like Hahnemann with brains full of intelligence and knowledge. His theory of osteopathy says that the body possesses the power for self-healing and self-maintenance. When doctors of his era believed in giving opium and whisky to eliminate pains, he went against this stream. Osteopathy relieves the patients of pain and aches by putting into use the art and science of manipulations. Fingers do these manipulations by pressure, by slow and soft touching and finding exact nerves and bone to manipulate them to their actual position. This therapy is not new to Indians. There is a reference of this type of therapy in Ayurveda. 'Sushruta Samhita' the ancient book written by Sushruta, the student of Dhanvantri has written about 'Asthi chikitsa' (Bones treatment). Manipulation is one of the oldest techniques used for healing ills of the body. Even today in our villages, towns and cities, we have bonesetters or 'Pehlwans' (wrestlers doing this job of bone setting through massages, bandaging, oil applications and exact manipulations). It is nothing but 'finger surgery' of our 'Pehlwans' although this has been made outdated by the advance methods propagated by Dr. Still.

One must remember that Hippocrates, the pioneer of medicine, was the one who introduced manipulation of joints, bones and spine of patients. He was actually practicing this therapy on his patients. Today the medical world does not recognize this sort of therapy called osteopathy although it is in vogue in the US and Britain. If I am not wrong, there is a London College of Osteopathy in London, which imparts training and course of 14 months to post graduate students of medicine. Moreover, there are six colleges of osteopathy in USA.

During the times when Hahnemann and Still were busy finding new concepts, we must acknowledge that this was the era when a lot more was contributed to the advancement of medical science. Pasteur was making studies on 'germ' theory, Lister was working on theory of antisepsis and Virchow conducting experiments on the theory of physiology. It was during the end of nineteenth century and beginning of twentieth century that use of Diphtheria antitoxins, X-ray machine and Blood pressure reading instrument were invented.

It is also amazing to think that both Hahnemann and Still had somewhat similar ideas. They both believed that the body is a complete unit and it not possible for one part of the unit to be sick without affecting other parts of the body. Both of them believed in the treatment of the body as a whole and that body's self-mechanism (Hahnemann's vital force) should be recognized and normalized (says Still).

"Man is a wonderful creation of God. It is a self sufficient and self-maintaining machine. This machine would run smoothly and look after itself", says Still.

"The power of nature frequently accomplishes wonderful, quick and beautiful cures. Serious illnesses often get better of themselves. Also in chronic affections, this marvelous power of healing asserts itself", says Hahnemann (Life of Hahnemann by Rosa W. Hobhouse published by M/s B.Jain Publishers).

In reference with our subject, if we examine other systems of medicines, it is more tilting towards the non-medicine side than induction of medicines for neck pains. We have therapies like Acupuncture, Acupressure, Osteopathy, Chiropractic, Reiki, Naturopathy, Hydrotherapy, Hypnotism, Yoga, Meditation, Physiotherapy and Homoeopathy. All these systems believe in no medicines or little medicines. I have not much of experience in other therapies but Homoeopathy and natural healing via exercise or manipulation or Yoga, as someone would like to state, are certainly beneficial to remove neck pains.

It will, therefore, be very much beneficial if the wisdom and intelligence of both the therapies, Homoeopathy and Osteopathy are applied, the neck pain or pains in the back can be eliminated in no time. But this is only well said than done. It is very difficult to find a person who should be well conversant with both the therapies, especially, when Osteopathy is not even known in many parts of the world.

Dr. Krishan Murari Modi, a qualified graduate of medicines and osteopathy from London, writer of a wonderful book on osteopathy, is a well-known osteopath of India. In his book,

'Cure, Aches and Pains through Osteopathy' he claims to have cured many patients by osteopathy. According to him, the spine, the birthplace of all pains, is like a "Sitar" (musical instrument). It has to be handled very carefully to produce positive notes and tunes dear to the ears. Sitar cannot be learnt overnight. It needs practice and one has to master it before displaying the art. It is true that the art of manipulation cannot be learnt from books.

'It is the part of the therapy mentioned in orthopedic text books', says Dr. Modi, 'Very few practitioners try to use them under general anesthesia and many do not use them at all. Few of them frankly admit, "As we do not know how to manipulate we do not use them in our practice, neither we teach them to our students". Osteopaths have the same legal status as medical practitioners in America. America is its birthplace and there are six osteopathic medical colleges in US where four years of medical course and one year internship is prescribed. In America only qualified osteopaths can practice whereas in Britain, any professional can practice osteopathy.

What can be, then, alternative when one doctor expert in both osteopathy and homoeopathy is not available. Even people do not believe that such a person would be definitely curing the disease. The simple course adopted by the patients is to consult the nearest orthopedic consultant or the nearest physician and get the treatment. Going to a 'bone-setter' or a 'Pehalwan' is a matter of the past. Now whenever someone meets an accident and breaks the bone, the procedure is well known. No one goes to a 'bone-setter' to fix the same. One can see his broken bone on x-ray film before the treatment and after plastering or operations, the bone can be again seen fixed. In the case of a neck pain or pain in the back, nothing can be done when x-ray etc.

show regular correct features of the spine and no deformity. What can a doctor prescribe except pain killing medicines and some local applicants or hot bandage to soothe the muscles. It is here that the patient is drawn towards alternative therapies like acupressure, homoeopathy etc. Yoga is always given the last preference because of the physical strains (so called) one has to undergo and the time taken for conducting the exercises. Yes, I have seen that homoeopathy clicks a number of times giving relief to the patient but again after some time, the patient is back to square one. It is here that the blame goes to the therapy used. There is no reason why a therapy should fail, be it any therapy. It is the other side. The patient has not tried to follow the instructions of the doctor in regards to change of life style, the sitting posture and other directions given. The sitting, lying, weight lifting and work-seat postures are very important. If those are defied with and wrong postures are continued, the neck pain or the backache can return.

It is not the nature of therapy or the treatment, which is curing the patient of the neck pain but it is the right measures adopted after the first treatment becomes successful. We are talking of osteopathy and homoeopathy here to cure neck pain. Let us leave this topic and come to the exact subject of neck pain. To understand its disease process and pathology, its nature and complications, we have to know something about the structure of neck and connected organs.

CONTENTS

1
PART

CHAPTER 1

THE SPINE

E VERY BODY knows what a spine is? There is a prov-
erb concerning spine. If someone is coward, gets de-
feated easily or is unable to stand the hardships of life, people
call him a spineless or gutless fellow. Man is a vertebrate. This
means that man has a backbone called spine. Spine has a series
of small irregular bones linked together and yet can move of
their own. *There are twenty-three such links or segments which are
mobile.* Spine is the backbone of our structure in which there is
a spinal cord, a 45-centimeter long and one-centimeter thick
livewire. This cord is like a telephone wire over which the mes-
sages of the brain and body are interconnected. To accomplish
this job, there are 31 pairs of nerves branching out from the
cord. Some of the nerves of the cord convey message of the
brain direct to the muscles and that too in split seconds. Suppose the sole of your feet gets a thorn pinch, within no time
your hand reaches the spot to pull out the throne. In split seconds, the sole nerves send a message of its grievance and the
hand reaches the spot spontaneously. What a wonderful mecha-

UNDERSTANDING A HEALTHY SPINE

Cervical curve

Thoracic curve

Lumbar curve

Abdominal muscles

Buttock muscles

Quadriceps muscles

Hamstring muscles

The back's three natural curves are correctly aligned when the ears, shoulders, and hips are in a straight line.

nism is of sensory and motor nerves to transmit the order from foot to brain and from brain to the hand muscles. The spine is like a central pole of a tent without which the tent cannot stand erect and will fall down. It is the spine, which holds the head and makes it swivel sidewise and up-down. Again it is the spine, which supports the weight of the body.

Although we shall be discussing about the neck and back pain in detail in the book later, yet it is worthwhile to state that the spine is very sensitive and it can also bring pain of its own without any apparent physical reason or inflammation etc. If a person is worried and under great tension or emotionally upset for a longer duration, the result in the body is a dull backache. Mind it there is no physical reason for getting a backache. The effects of any nature on the brain are bound to reflect on the spine. Worry and emotions put a stress on the spine and then tighten the sensitive muscles of the spine. This results in a 'tired spine' giving a dull pain in the back.

Spine lies in the central axis of our skeleton and its shape is like a chain of bones just like a reel of film. It is a marvel of engineering, created by God to see that you stand erect and straight. The wonder of the wonder is that the spine itself is not straight while it makes you stand straight. The vertebrae in the spine do not remain in the same position i.e. the vague 'S' position unless there is no movement of the body. There is always slight movement in the body even while sleeping and turning sides and hence the vertebrae settle in different position when one is sitting, standing, holding weight, leaning against some pillar, bending and lifting something, lying down and walking. There will be slight temporary changes in the curves of spine during the day-time when one is working due to varying activities. The normal motions of the spine are flexion (bending forward, backward and sideways) and rotation or turning. The beauty is that in spite of small movements of the vertebrae, the flexibility is enormous and the spine has the capability of larger amount of free movement. The example of this heavy amount of free movement can be witnessed by the performance of a dancer or a gymnast.

VERTEBRAL COLUMN

- The neck of the spine has *seven cervical vertebrae. Cervical means pertaining to neck or cervix and vertebrae is bony segment of the spinal column.*

- On the upper back of the body lie *twelve thoracic vertebrae. Thoracic means pertaining to chest.* This area is also called *dorsal spine.* This area of the back is almost trouble free and it causes very rare pains, leave aside traumas. The reason can be well understood. There is not much of movement here in this part of the spine and our ribs are connected to it.

- At the lower back, the spine has *five lumbar vertebrae. Lumbar means pertaining to loins or lower part of the back.* These vertebrae stand most of the weight of the body. In many cases of back pain, it is the fourth and fifth lumbar vertebrae, which is the trouble spot or the pain emitting station.

- The lowest back area has *five sacral vertebrae. Sacral is area of sacrum.* These five segments are fused together to make coccyx below which we have the coccygeal bone formed by four rudimentary coccyx bones. Coccyx is the tail of the spine.

CURVES OF SPINE

It is just like a vague 'S'. If the spine is viewed from side, one can see four graceful curves in a healthy spine. Let us discuss about the curves first.

- In the neck region or cervical, the curve of the spine is slightly forward or convex forward.

- In the chest region or thoracic from second to twelfth thoracic spine, the curve is concave forward or distinct backward curvature.

- In the lumbar region or abdominal area, it is again convex forward. The spine curves forward in this region.

- In the pelvic region, the spine has a backward swing. This pelvic curve goes from lumbo-sacral joint to the apex of the coccyx. The spine's concavity faces forward and downward.

VERTEBRAE

We have talked about vertebra. It is a body lying in front and really supports the weight of the body. Its posterior projection is called *neural arch. It is this neural canal through which passes the spinal cord.* In this arc are six parts called pedicle, pair of transverse processes, superior articular process, inferior articular process, spinous process and laminae. We shall not go into details of the peculiar functions of these parts because our aim is to use less of medical terms to avoid confusion for the mass readers of the book.

It is worth mentioning here that the body of each vertebra fits well with that of one above it and the one below it. Each vertebra has a close link with the other and yet a small resilient disc of cartilage separates them. This disc serves as shock absorber. About disc, we shall discuss later. In the vertebral processes, every top and bottom of a vertebra has a little flat surface. This surface is called facet of the vertebra. Actually facet joints are the true joints of the spine. (Please see a separate heading, posterior joints below)

Vertebrae of the spine are well connected and *joined with an entangled or intricate series of muscles, ligaments and tendons to make the whole setup a structure easily flexible and moveable. It is strong enough to stand jerks on the spine and gives a support to the head, shoulders and the trunk besides holding the ribs at the top and pelvis at the bottom. You must have observed in the grain market that laborers carry a quintal of grain in the gunny bag on their backs without difficulty and load or unload the same in trucks or vehicles. They are actually handing over this load to their spines. It is this wonderful spine that is capable of carrying loads and pressures of hundreds of kilograms without giving even a little cry of pain. Personally I have checked with the laborers of 'Anaj Mandi' to find out the secret of their carrying so much of load and still never report any pains. As a matter of fact, I sit in Arya Samaj hospital that is very near to this Mandi and the laborers of this Mandi make frequent visits to this charitable hospital for minor ailments. To my surprise, no laborer comes to me for muscular pains in their

---

*There are intervertebral joints, which consist of muscles, nerves, intervertebral foreman, anterior joint having disc and posterior joint made of facet joints.

body. The reason for such a condition is that they take about 50 gms of 'Channa' with 'Gurh' every day.

THE POSTERIOR, ANTERIOR JOINTS AND LIGAMENTS OF THE SPINE

We have already discussed about various joints of the spine above but the actual joints of the spine are posterior joints. The whole of the movement and its variety of movement has a base upon the direction and shape of facet joints. These facet joints have thin, elastic and loose articular covering which is quite dense. In the cervical spine, the covering is larger and loose. (Please note that we are not discussing much about lumbar and thoracic regions). Each facet joint is supplied by a nerve, which goes to two adjoining joints. This means that each joint takes nerve supply from two segments. Every vertebra has two superior and two inferior facet joints. There is intra-articular substance called menisci, which is quite elastic and acts as a cushion. This has a rich blood supply and nerve supply. *In the region of cervical, the superior facet joints are angled upwards to about forty-five degrees and that is the reason of free flexion and rising or extension of neck.* More than flexion, extension can be done and of course bending the neck or rotating the neck are both combined. Superior facet joints are more oblique in the thoracic region. They are supported by ribs and the body and have restricted movements due to the direction of the facet joints. So here, the rotation is of greater range than the extension or flexion. In the thoracic region, lateral bending cannot be done due to the restriction of ribs and sternum. In comparison, if you see the lumbar spine, one can conduct rotation and side bending to some extent because of freeness from the ribs and sternum.

ROLE OF LIGAMENTS

Coming to *ligaments*, it can be said that *the role of the ligaments is to hold the bones together and also allow some limited movements to the vertebrae.* In other words, the vertebrae are held together by ligaments to make a spine. So they can be called or considered joints in some way because they form a sort of capsule around the joints. Ligaments do the so-called harmonious movement of the spine. We can also say that there are a number of ligaments spread from second cervical to the first sacral. As a matter of fact, anterior and posterior ligaments join whole of the vertebrae body. Ligaments have a wonderful capacity of flexibility and stretching capability because of their elastic structure. When due to some external trauma, unwanted exercise or even moderate exercise having prolonged stretching, or by sudden force, the ligament is stretched or torn; the pain is felt at the neck due to degeneration of disc. Degeneration of disc means that the spine at the place of degeneration is stressed and stress or the accentuation means added pain. What happens is that due to abnormal movement of say neck, the blood vessels supplying blood to the spinal cord get blocked. Blood's scarcity makes the cells dead. This condition would require only operation. There is more than one factor leading to operation. This condition is very common and it can be treated if diagnosed in time. About the torn condition of the ligaments, the doctors can only make an estimate based upon experience and touch because *the ligaments are not seen in the X-ray reports.*

ANTERIOR LIGAMENTS

On the anterior surface of the vertebrae, there is a long,

strong fibrous group of *longitudinal ligaments, anterior.* These ligaments are coupled with margins of vertebral body and disc. These ligaments are broad at the level of disc and narrow at the level of the body. If these ligaments are torn, there will be edema and hemorrhage. Whenever this occurs, one should give sufficient time of rest to the back and neck for its self-repairs. If these ligaments are stretched for a longer period, there is likelihood of pain especially in the area of neck, which we are discussing.

POSTERIOR LIGAMENTS

Within vertebral canal and attached to the vertebral body are attached *posterior longitudinal ligaments.* They are coupled with the intervertebral disc firmly and also with the vertebral body forming a bridge over it. The main purpose of this ligament is to strengthen the position of disc posteriorly but it has a vital role to play in disc protrusion. It is the resistance of this ligament that holds back the protrusion of disc. Most of the times, this happens in the case of backache in lumbar region and hence we shall not go into details. Similarly we shall not go into deep details of other types of ligaments like ligamentum flavum, supra-spinous and inter-spinous ligaments.

MUSCLES

The motor apparatus of our body has vital and active participant in the form of muscles. It is the contraction of muscles that produce various movements. From the function point of view, muscles can be organized into two groups, voluntary and involuntary.

Voluntary muscles are striated muscles tissue and get contracted by the will of the man. (Striated means marked with furrows or stripped muscles subject to control by will). Striated are those included in the muscles of head, trunk, extremities like skeletal muscles and muscles of internal organs like tongue, larynx etc. Voluntary muscles are called *skeletal* also. All form of conscious movement like running over a flight of stairs and re-actions like reflexes are by these muscles. Voluntary muscles are distributed throughout the body, making up a large portion. They are like springs attached with different parts of skeleton and control the movement of different bones.

Involuntary muscles are nonstriated muscle tissue and are found in the walls of internal organs, blood vessels and the skin. The contraction of these muscles is not controlled by the will of man. The guts and bladder are two examples of these muscles. In involuntary muscles, each fibre is a spindly cell. These are not under the conscious control of brain. They are responsible for the muscular contractions needed in workings like rhythmic squeezing of the intestines to move food, and digesting food.

Some scholars say that there is a third type of muscle in the body. It is the cardiac muscles, which makes up the main bulk of the heart. Heart muscles are not controlled by the will but contain striated muscle tissue with a special structure. Their fibres are short and thick and form a dense mesh. Involuntary muscles are also called *smooth* muscles also because they look very smooth under a microscope.

There are more than four hundred skeletal muscles in the

human organism in adults and they make up about two-fifths of the total body weight.

Some of the muscles really act upon the spine and also help in the movement of neck and back. Muscles keep the spine steady. Their main job is to produce sort of extension, lateral bending and rotation of the neck and body. Muscles also help maintain the posture. Of course, the more of help is from abdominal muscles. Weakness of muscles may result in deformity of spine (scoliosis).

Sudden trauma or movement may produce imbalanced distribution of forces on the vertebral joints and result in compression of spinal cord and muscle spasm. When the muscles are weak, the strain is more on ligaments and the joints and the weak muscles are the results of bad postures.

ROLE OF MUSCLES PLAY IN NECK PAIN

Like all other tissues, muscular tissue contains the property of excitability. *Excitability is the ability to respond to stimulation and become active.* Unlike other tissues, the main job of the muscular tissue is contraction, which other tissues do not perform. *Contraction is shortening.* A contracting muscles will become short and thick but there will be no change in its volume and the beauty is that muscles can do work when they contract. It is the nerve impulse reaching the muscles from the central nervous system (along motor nerves) which makes the muscles contracted. We have already discussed that the contraction of striated muscles are controlled consciously and smooth muscles move involuntarily.

Muscles do have the property of tensility. *Tensility is the ability to stretch* to some limit. When the reason producing the stretching is no more or disappears, the muscles return to the former state. This property of returning to original state in muscles is called *elasticity*.

INTERVERTEBRAL FORAMAN

As the name suggests, the intervertebral *foramen is a short canal* lodged between contiguous vertebrae. It is oval in form but may change its shape with the mobility of the inter-vertebral joint. In cervical spine, it is slightly to the front side as compared to the dorsal and lumbar spine. The spinal cord passes through it and it contains enough blood capillaries making vascular pocket. There may be a sort of compression or irritation in the V. foramen on account of degeneration of disc, rupture of disc or posterior profusion of disc and cause lot of pain and muscular weakness. The conditions more likely to occur are lumbago and sciatica.

DISCS

The vague 'S' like shape of the spine is made to bear the jolts and shocks and acts like shock absorber for the back. Discs are the tools to keep the vertebrae together. The importance of the discs in the spine can be guessed by the fact that they constitute one fourth of the whole length of spine. Discs absorb the shock as if they are made of rubber or has some hidden hydraulic system. Sometimes man is unable to explain the mystery of how or why of human body construction. The elastic properties of the discs and the spine cannot be explained in words. By now it is clear that plate in between each pair of vertebrae is called *Disc*. Disc has three parts, the end plate part, the peripheral part named as *annulus fibrosus* and a central part called *nucleus pulposus*. In healthy condition, the vertebrae have very smooth edges but after the discs get degenerated, the edges of the vertebral body start having friction against each other or get rubbed against each other. This condition is against the normal smooth rubbing and hence the cause of pain. With this rubbing continuous, the edges of the body develop bony spikes. These spikes are sharp and pointed. And if these spikes pinch the nerve roots, the pain of the neck is radiated to the arms. If the spike entangles with nerves and compress the nerves of the cord, even paralysis of the legs cannot be ruled out.

Disc is given its nourishment by synovial fluid and if a part of disc wears out, it remains alive in the joint cavity. The cartilage contains no blood supply or nerve system and hence it is slow to act or give impression of pain when the back meets an accident. The pain, therefore, is slow to come when the cartilage is damaged. Immediate pain will be there if the adjoining sensitive muscles are damaged. The beauty is that while cartilage gets swelling due to forced activity of the accident but with no nerve or blood supply, there is no pain. The swelling is a very slow process. In such cases, sufficient rest is needed, which people do not follow and the swelling increases with movements continued. Disc also has a quality of sponge and can absorb fluid or diffuse out its own fluid content. There is always a change occurring in the consistency of the discs.

Disc is very common term and most of the back-sufferers know what is slip disc. When this disc gets dislocated or tilted or gets out of alignment due to some accident or other reasons, it is called *slip disc*. The discs are cushions plated by a thick film (cartilage) of jelly like substance. When the jelly like substance is eroded or leaked due to some rupture, vehicle accident or a fall, there is acute pain_and further complications start. With the film coating of the jelly like substance over the disc missing or leaking out, the discs are likely to make friction with the adjoining nerves. The outcome is spasms of muscles. Under this condition, the person bends forward and gets some relief. Bending forward means removing of friction. The other worse effect of the ruptured disc is the irritation of the sciatic nerve. This will bring pain all along the nerve length extending to legs.

It is uncommon that a disc on the neck area ruptures. If it does, the pain radiates down the shoulder and arms. If the muscles of neck get stretched or inflamed, the result is a stiff neck. Cervical spine has a very small area of vertebrae but their body and facet joints stand a large ball weighing about 12 lbs. head of the man. We know that the head is balanced on two small facets, which are small as nails and yet these have a flexible mobility in all directions. The joint is strong that it can carry a weight ten times the weight of the head, which it carries always. The support of the head is also by two upper cervical vertebrae.

As and when some degenerative changes take place in the middle age group persons, *bulging of the disc material* may come up in any direction and it will bring a pull on the ligaments during weight bearing. Under these circumstances, new bone formation could occur under this periosteal lift and after some time, *osteophytes* (bony outgrowth) appear. The osteophytes then restrict the mobility and ligaments are hardened. It is not a painful condition in most of the cases.

SPINAL CORD

The spinal cord is a compact mass of gray and white matter in which a group of nerves run in the canal formed by the hole in the bodies of the vertebrae. The *gray matter* is in the center of the cord whereas the *white matter* is outside. If the horizontal section of the spine is seen, the gray matter can be seen in the form of a butterfly with two anterior projections, the ventral horns and two posterior projections, the dorsal horns. The ventral horns are wider than the dorsal horns. The gray matter surrounding the spinal canal is called *gray commissure.* The ventral horns have motor nerve cells, while the dorsal horns contain internuncial nerve cells which effect communication between other nerve cells, for example between sensory and motor nerve cells. The sensory nerve cells are located not in the spinal cord, but along the sensory nerves, in the intervertebral foramina where they form accumulations called spinal ganglia. Both the motor and sensory nerves run from the brain to enervate different parts of the body. The spinal cord is surrounded by laminae (a thin layer, scale or plate, usually of bone) from each side of vertebra. The laminae of vertebrae make the spinal canal through which the cord passes downwards. It is this canal, which protects the cord from external injuries. We make lot of movements of neck when seeing sidewise, up or down but the spinal cord is always well protected during the various movements. So far as the nerve roots are within the canal, there is no harm to them but they come out of the canal at each level of the vertebrae on either side. At this very juncture of their exposure, the nerve roots should not be compressed or get pinched during normal movements of the neck. This is the reason why doctors advise neck movement exercises to be done slowly and not abruptly.

Whenever we do some hard work, carry weight, bend ourselves in normal range of bending and do jumping or in other words when our movements include flexing and extensional curving, there has to be thrust and pressure on the spine and the cord. Here in such cases, the thrust is intermittent and does not cause abnormal or notable harm to the cord. But on the other hand, if this flexing and extensive curving is continued for some months or years without taking much of care to change pattern and postures of working, the spurs (bony spikes) form on the edges of vertebral bodies. *Spur literally means the projecting portion.* We have talked about osteophytes in the above description of disc. *Osteophytes and spurs are one and the same thing.* Once the spurs form, more of damage is caused. Having a persistent pressure from the disc-edges sides, the cord is compressed and the result may be a paralysis or a constant weakness with or without pain in the arms in case of vertebra of the cervical/thoracic region and a paralysis in the legs if the vertebra is of lumbar/coccyx region. When the X-ray report of the spine gives a picture of spurs, the patient has to be careful.

THE JOB OF SPINAL CORD

The spinal cord has two functions, conducting nerve impulses (excitation) and reflex activity. The spinal cord has a communication network through nerve fibres, its nervous pathways, with various parts of the brain and through spinal nerves with organs like skin, muscles and blood vessels etc. The cord has two types of nervous pathways, the ascending, which is sensory and descending, which is motor. The spinal nerves have also two kinds of nerve fibre, sensory and motor.

The nerve impulses communicated to the spinal cord from the periphery (organs), along sensory fibres of the spinal nerves, are then conducted along the ascending nervous pathways to the brain. The various parts of the brain perceive these excitations. For instance, the excitation coming up in the receptors of the skin, when stimulated, is transmitted to the cerebral cortex. This is how the sensations such as cold, heat, pain etc. arise in the cortex.

The nerve impulses are transmitted from the brain to the spinal cord along the descending pathways and thence along motor fibres of the spinal nerve to the periphery i.e. organs. These impulses or excitations change the state of various organs. For instance, they produce contraction of skeletal muscles, voluntary retention of the urine and faeces etc.

When we talk of *reflex activity of the spinal cord,* it is interesting. The spinal cord has the reflex centers of muscular activity. Each segment of the spinal cord is related with certain group of muscles.

The cervical segment of the spinal cord, the concern of our subject, contains the centers of reflex movement of the diaphragm, muscles of the neck, the shoulder girdle and upper extremities.

The thoracic segments contain the centers of the trunk muscles.

The lumbar and sacral segments contain the centers of the pelvic muscles and muscles of the lower extremities.

The spinal cord has also the centers of certain other reflexes. For example, the centers of perspiration and vasomotor are located in the thoracic and lumbar divisions and the centers of urination, defecation and activity of sex organs are located in the sacral division.

It is known that all muscles are continuously under the state of tension (tone). The muscles, tendons, ligaments and joint capsules have sensory nerve endings called *proprioceptors.* These receptors are stimulated when one changes the position of muscles, joints and ligaments, which means when one is under some activity. The excitation here is communicated along sensory nerves to the spinal cord and then to motor nerves and further to the muscles. All this result in continuous state of tension (tone) for the muscles. In case of any damage to the spinal cord due to some accident or otherwise, there are many changes in the function of the cord. If the nervous pathways in various parts of the body are injured, their sensitivity is lost, voluntary muscular contraction is impaired (under paralytic condition). Damage to centers of the spinal cord generally amounts to loss of reflexes.

THE NECK

This book is mainly with a purpose to describe and treat cervical spondylosis and hence it would be in the right direction if muscles and **fasciae* are also described.

---

* A *Fascia* is a thick or thin but dense band of connective tissue, which binds a muscle or group of muscles. In the various regions of the body, fasciae differ a lot in thickness and they are usually named after the location of the muscles such as fasciae of shoulder, of the neck, of the forearm etc. Fasciae are also connected and continuous with the other regions of the body and hence form a sort of tissue sheath to prevent sideward displacement of muscles.

The muscles of the neck are of four kinds or groups in general:

- *The platysma myoides muscle* is a thin, broad band of muscle situated under the skin on the lateral surface of neck and lowers the corners of the mouth.

- *The sternocleidomastoid muscle* is the largest muscle of the neck and it has extension from the clavicle and sternum to the mastoid process. The function of the muscle is to bend the head to the side and turning the face to the opposite side. On contraction of muscle on the both sides, the head is thrown back.

- *The muscles situated above and below the hyoid bone* lower the mandible and if the mandible is fixed, raise the hyoid bone and the larynx. These movements are initiated while swallowing and chewing.

- *Deep muscles of the neck* are the three muscles, (anterior, middle and posterior) called scalenus muscles. These muscles have their origin in the cervical vertebrae and their place of insertion is on the first and second ribs. These muscles raise the ribs and thereby participate in inhalation. There is a space between the anterior and middle muscles called the scalenus interspaced which contains blood vessels and nerves.

FASCIAE OF THE NECK

Our neck has *three fasciae, superficial, middle and deep.*

As the names indicate, these three layers of muscles above and below the hyoid bone form the capsule of the sub-maxillary gland and are connected with the veins of the neck. It is the deep fascia of the neck, which covers deep muscles of the neck and the cervical part of the neck. Excessive stretch of these muscles sometimes becomes the reason for stiff neck and pain.

CHAPTER 2

SPONDYLITIS

A BRIEF ACCOUNT of the spinal cord and its local lesions is given here to have a peep into our subject just for knowledge sake. *The compression of the spinal cord* is one of the causes for pains in cervical region. In compression, the lumen of the spinal canal is reduced in a small part of its vertical extent and the spinal cord is injured at this point either directly by pressure or indirectly by interference with its vascular supply. All the extra medullary lesions of the spinal cord come under this heading except acute inflammation of the membranes. Compression of the spinal cord can be divided into two parts, slow compression and rapid compression. In slow compression, the reason is tuberculous spinal caries, vertebral tumors, meningeal tumors and cysts besides rare causes like leukemia, aneurysm, syphilitic caries and spondylitis deformans etc. In case the cervical spondylitis persists for a longer time and is not getting cured after lot of medication, it is always better to get clinical and laboratory tests done so that proper diagnosis is done for above diseases.

COMMON SPINE AND DISK PROBLEMS

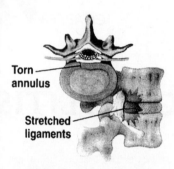

Torn annulus

Stretched ligaments

Torn annulus. A sudden movement may cause a tiny tear in an annulus. Nearby ligaments may stretch.

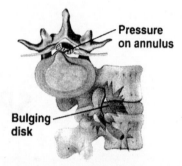

Pressure on annulus

Bulging disk

Bulging disk. As a disk wears out, the nucleus begins to bulge into the annulus.

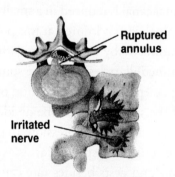

Ruptured annulus

Irritated nerve

Ruptured disk. As a disk ruptures, its nucleus can squeeze out and irritate a nerve.

In some cases of cervical spondylitis, the pain and impairment of movement of the cervical joints commonly accompany the ordinary types of *non-specific infective arthritis*. In some other cases, the whole vertebrae may be involved and marked fixation of the spine ensues, sometimes with deformity resulting in the bowing commonly seen in the old people. This is *spondylitis deformans*. It is due to osteophytic changes and the bony outgrowth.

The most important step is first to find out the cause of the infection and the pain in the cervical regions, which has given rise to all above diseases. All cervical pains and stiffness of neck etc. are not on account of bad postures or exposures etc.

A careful and complete clinical examination should be made to discover any possible source of infection, including X-ray examination.

LUMBAR SPONDYLITIS, DORSAL SPONDYLITIS

When we talk of the term spondylitis, we have three types. *Lumbar spondylitis, Dorsal spondylitis and Ankylosing spondylitis.*

Lumbar spondylitis is stated to be next to importance to the cervical spondylitis. In this case, the reason is same i.e. degenerative changes in the lumbar region of the spine. The pain thus caused is called lumbago, a well-known definition for medical students. In general public, *it is called backache*.

*Dorsal spondylitis is the very less important than the cervical or lumbar spondylitis because of the fact that it occurs

---

*Dorsal means pertaining to back, thoracic area or posterior part of spine.

COMMON SPINE AND DISK PROBLEMS

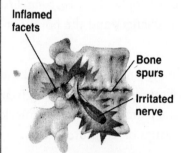

Inflamed facets

Bone spurs

Irritated nerve

Arthritis. As disks wear out over time, bone spurs form. These growths can irritate nerves and inflame facets.

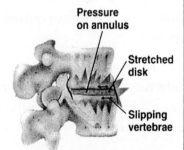

Pressure on annulus

Stretched disk

Slipping vertebrae

Instability. As a disk stretches, the vertebrae slip back and forth. This can put pressure on the annulus.

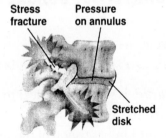

Stress fracture   **Pressure on annulus**

Stretched disk

Spondylolisthesis. A crack (stress fracture) can develop in a vertebra. This may put pressure on the annulus, stretch the disk, and irritate nerves.

very less. We have already stated that this area of back is well supported by the ribs and shoulder bones and less prone to aches. Here also the degenerative changes occur in the intervertebral discs of the vertebrae in the thoracic region.

ANKYLOSING SPONDYLITIS*

Before we discuss about cervical spondylosis, it is better to know about ankylosing spondylitis. *Ankylosing means stiffness.* It is a progressive inflammatory arthritis, which through calcification of the ligaments attached to the vertebrae forms an abnormal immobility and consolidations of the joints. With the synovitis** of the vertebrae joints, this disease starts. This is a serious beginning and if the disease is not controlled in time through proper medication, the spine becomes stiff and looks like a bamboo. (Bamboo spine or poker spine is the name given by doctors). The bamboo is never seen as straight erected on the ground of its original plant and so is the case of *bamboo spine.* The spine gets a little bent over and the person affected becomes hunch-backed. In bamboo spine cases, the vertebrae mainly affected are those of the lumbar and the lower cervical regions.

REASONS

Most affected persons of ankylosing spondylitis are from the age group of 17 to 40 years and men are about ten times more prone to this disease than women. The reason of this type of disease is obscure. In some cases there are symptoms of some kind of infection or an infective process though so far no part of

Two vertebrae and a disk

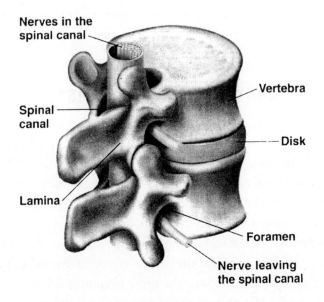

Nerves in the spinal canal

Spinal canal

Lamina

Vertebra

Disk

Foramen

Nerve leaving the spinal canal

Top view of a vertebra and a disk

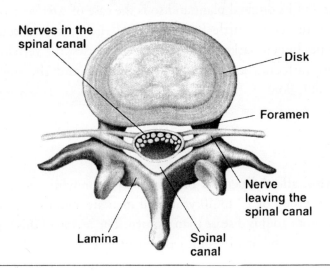

Nerves in the spinal canal

Disk

Foramen

Nerve leaving the spinal canal

Lamina

Spinal canal

the body is responsible for this infection. In few cases, it appears to be precipitated by an injury in the back. Some doctors have observed that persons having prostatitis or some other inflammatory lesions of the genito-urinary tracts get this disease of ankylosing spondylitis. *Speaking of Homoeopathy, we can say that the etiology of this disease pertains to familial (pertaining to family) cause and due to an inherited miasm.*

CLINICAL SIGNS AND PROGNOSIS

The start of the disease is stealthy or insidious with a sort of feeling that there is something wrong in the body or there may be slight fever. In about twenty five to thirty percent of cases, iritis*** may occur and this may occasionally be the first sign of the disease. Pain in the neck, muscle spasm and deformity are the later developments from ankylosis. Ankylosing spondylosis does not endanger the life by itself. Of course those who die of this disease normally develop some respiratory infection due to the reduced vital capacity resulting from the ankylosis of the costovertebral joints.

---

*In medical terms both spondylosis and spondylitis are same.

**Synovia is a lubricating fluid secreted in the joints of the bones and synovitis is the inflammation of synovial membrane.

***Iritis is inflammation of the iris. Iris is the colored layer of the eye, surrounding the pupil.

CHAPTER 3

CERVICAL SPONDYLOSIS OR NECK PAIN

CERVICAL SPONDYLOSIS is a condition pertaining to degenerative process caused by mainly two factors.

- Degeneration of the intervertebral discs with the formation of bony ridges running across the anterior surface of the neural canal.

- The formation of osteophytes from the neurocentral joints of Luscka, which project backwards into the intervertebral foramen.

We have many other reasons but basically we shall discuss here two important reasons of the cervical spondylosis.

- If there is a sudden stress or jerk in the neck area due to violent forward lurch as a result of some road traffic accident, this can give rise to the neck pain in the occipital, post-auricular regions, and in the upper part of the trapezius, and between the shoulder blades. Such an injury is called 'whip lash injury'. Since pain and muscle spasm in the lower cervical region is the result of movement in the painful joints, wearing a collar often relieves these symptoms.

■ If the reason is not an accident but compression of arteries and veins due to bony ridges on the anterior surface of the cord, the treatment has to be done by medicines and physiotherapy before resorting to surgery in some cases.

The torturing excruciating pain in the neck is really an unnerving one. In the modern type of living when the person is more dependent upon electronic gadgets having less of mobility, neck pain ranks high on the list of ailments, which a person is responsible to self-inflict. In the fashion we are following, work and work with no physical exercise in our daily routine, we are likely to have neck pain at one time or the other. The exception is with the villagers who are not prone to this type of neck pain. They do have neck pain but it is only due to carrying excessive load on their heads and due to strain as in the case of rural area inhabitants. During my thirty-five years of life spent in the villages and jungles, I have not come across villagers wearing neck collars or complaining of neck pains. As a matter of fact, we are ignoring our routine of physical exercises inherited from our elders or we can say that we are defying our evolutionary heritage and making ourselves sedentary human beings. The better part of our job is spent sitting at desks, at shops, in the car, driving and even eating or reading at home keeping bad postures. Such changes in our life-style have a negative impact on human physiology.

In short we can say that neck pain is the product of very fast life, mechanical routine, lack of exercise, bad postures, sitting or sleeping, and tensions besides the injuries. Neck pain is not due to one specific reason.

In the neck pain, the degenerative changes occur in the intervertebral discs leading to their rupture or prolapse. The disc between the 6th and 7th vertebrae is affected most of the times but discs between the 4th and 5th vertebrae or 5th and 6th vertebrae cannot be ruled out for affections. Actually it is the anatomical relation of the disc protrusions and osteophytic outgrowths to the nerve roots and spinal cord and varies from person to person.

Every other office-goer or businessman suffers from it one day or the other. It counts not much when it goes of its own or by very little medication or by means of massage etc. This way, it is harmless and occasional neck pain cannot be taken as a disease. It may be due to wrong postures and exposures to dry old wind etc. The problem comes when the pain is persistent for a longer time. This cannot be ignored because it is the cervical column, which has wider effect on your brain activities than the problems or pains in the other columns of our back i.e. dorsal or lumbar spine. The neck has to stand the weight of head and be mobile as well. It has no support of ribs or pelvis as in the case of dorsal and lumbar regions. The neck stands alone without any support of bones from the adjoining organs. It has its own blood supply through vertebral arteries and veins. These vessels are well guarded in transverse processes but produce complications when the neck is not mobile or some mechanical problems interfere in the working of neck. When we talk of mobility, it has to be thought over seriously.

FIVE THINGS TO IDENTIFY YOUR NECK PROBLEMS

- Mobility is the first thing that reminds that there is something wrong in the neck.

- The second thing is pain in the neck and adjoining areas.

- The third thing is persistent aching or stiffness along the spine from the base of neck.

- The fourth thing is sharp localized pain in the neck radiating to either to the shoulders or hands or the upper back.

- The fifth thing is that there is chronic ache in the neck area if it is not cared with.

We shall now discuss about the limitation of mobility of neck and the pains in general.

Mobility-limitation is one of the main problems in the neck pain. We know that there is always a process of wear and tear going on in the body. We eat and drink and the burden is on whole of body, the stomach, the abdomen, the connective digestive organs, the intestines and series of actions take place to digest the things eaten. Eating is a continued process and without it we cannot survive. The digestive machinery is always in use and anything in persistent use is likely to have wear and tear. With the growing age, there is a general wear and tear of bones too and neck bones or the cervical spine is no exception.

TYPES OF PAIN

The pain the cervical spine mostly occurs in the three lowest cervical vertebrae. The first symptom is that patient is unable to turn the head or look behind. The pain also radiates to the posterior part of head or down to the immediate back, between the two shoulders and to both the shoulders.

Some people have this pain not directly in the neck. The neck is stiff but the pain is between the two shoulder blades. Such people, mostly ladies, have also some sort of swelling in the lower part of the neck. This swelling is prominent till the pain lasts but with improvement of mobility of neck, both the swelling and pain are reduced.

Persons with swelling of the neck area may have a degeneration of the disc between the vertebral bodies, as one of the causes of swelling. This can be confirmed by the X-ray report and one can see osteophytes at the facet joint margins.

Osteophytes occupy the place over intervertebral foramen and become a tool to reduce its size, which is the actual reason for causing pressure on the cervical nerves. With this process undergoing, the *patient may feel tingling, numbness* and pricking sensation of nails or needles in the hands.

When the condition is as above, there is another noted symptom. *The neck muscles get tender and at times* patient feels as if there is no pain in proper neck area and the movement of the neck is also free although some cracking sound may be there at times.

Whenever there is some pain in the body, say head, the patient can pin-point the area of pain but in the case of neck pain,

POSTURE TO RELIEVE PAIN IN BRACHIAL NEURALGIA

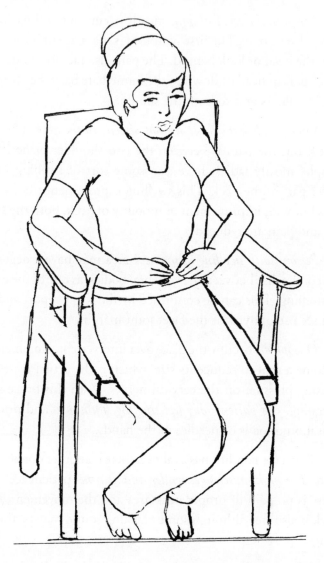

Sitting on armchair with body weight on elbows & forearms

it is difficult to pin-point an area with the tip of a finger. If there is pain with difficult mobility of the neck, it should be considered that whole of spine is affected and not only the neck area. In such a case, the pressure put on any area of spine should produce pain. This is true because spine is a single unit interconnected with all the three areas of the back including cervical, dorsal and lumbar-coccyx. The area of pain can be anywhere because of spinal integrated form and pathology can be anywhere in the intervertebral disc or posterior joints. By putting pressure on one area of the spine, we cannot determine the exact area of affection and hence it is advisable that X-ray should be taken to find out the exact location and nature of disease.

BRACHIALGIA

Brachial means pertaining to arms and brachialgia is pain in the arms. *Brachial neuralgia is the second phase of cervical spondylitis.* In many cases of neck pain, the arms become painful and the pain shoots down to one of the arms with numbness and tingling sensation. The irritation of the nerve roots emerging between second thoracic vertebrae and fourth cervical is the cause for brachialgia. With this as the main reason, *the other causes are pressure of the disc on the nerve root and inflammation of the nerve sheath or tissue contained in intervertebral foramen.*

One cannot rule out the bone involvement in a variable manner in some cases of brachialgia. The pain in the arm can be in whole of arm or localized at some place. In case of localized pain, it is felt only when some pressure is put. The type of pain can be severe or mild. The movement of the arm makes the patient cry with pain whereas keeping the arm still decreases the pain. In some patients, the pain is relieved when the patient puts his arms behind his neck or head. The chief complaint of the patient is stiffness of the neck. Brachialgia and pain in the shoulder blades are usual accompaniments. This stiffness when uncared for and with repeated attacks becomes the reason for protrusion of bones below neck area in the back. In such cases, the disc starts paining, movement of neck is restricted and the pain radiates towards upper limbs in accordance with the site of nerve pressure.

The best way to find out the brachialgia is as follows:

- Traction of the neck gives relief.

- If the lower part of the neck is painful, its movement, side-wise and up down, will increase the pain and could lead to numbness in the arm.

- There is weakness felt in the head and sometimes the patient, while in sitting posture, holds his head with his hands as if the weight of the head is intolerable for the neck.

- While lying down on the bed, there is restriction of even turning the head because it is painful and patient has to support his head.

CRACKING SOUND IN THE NECK

Some patients come to the doctor complaining that they do not have pains in the neck except on some occasions when they slip out of their pillows or place their heads or necks in some awkward position for a long time during sleep. Such patients get free of pains once some pain killer tablets are taken or some rest or massage is given to the neck. They come to doctors not to narrate this phenomenon of pain but they state a different problem of production of *some noise of cracking in the neck.* Those who have this cracking sound while turning the head get afraid and come to the doctor for a solution but there are some patients who do not bother about it and take pleasure in doing this act of cracking.

It is just like persons who make a click at their finger joints by pulling or bending the fingers and find pleasure. I have observed that persons having *abnormal and long necks* have this complaint most commonly. Those who are stout and short-necked do not have this problem. Although there is no fixed reason for the neck sound on turning yet some experts believe that it is because less of support from the bones of shoulders to the head. The area of neck stands aloof with the weight of head on it. The cracking sound mostly comes when the person crosses forty years of age. If ageing is the reason, the possibility of wear and tear of the bones cannot be ruled out but in such cases, there should not be cracking sound on turning. The set-up of bones is same as in the adulthood and only changes are the thinning or thickening of bones. The structure remains the same. If the neck structure is defective, say it is bent to one side or both thick and thin at places, there is a scope for bones to give cracking sound, when moved.

Another reason of cracking is self-made abnormality. This means a sort of accident to the neck area, which in turn might *produce some sort of vacuum* between the joints. However, there is no doubt that such cracking noise on the movement of neck is not an abnormal thing and harmless provided there is no pain. Noises in the knee joints are also common and people come to doctors for knowing the reason. Here again, if the noises are painless, there is no harm.

This is the medical theory but do Homoeopaths ignore this very symptom of noises in the joints? I am sure no Homoeopath ignores this very symptom. There are a number of remedies for cracking of knee-joints. This is an internal matter of the Homoeopath while he is in the process of selecting a remedy.

The duty of the doctor is that the painless cracking sound in the neck area should be described and told as harmless when a patient comes for this very clarification.

MUSCULAR FATIGUE

One of the reasons for cervical spondylosis is muscular fatigue, which has not been touched in our description about muscles.

Muscles in the human body are never completely relaxed even in the state of rest. This is one side of the picture. On the other side, muscles cannot work infinitely. During prolonged and uninterrupted work in a bad posture, the muscles gradually loose their working capacity. *Such a state is known as muscular fatigue.* In the case of muscular fatigue, the strength of muscular contraction decreases and the contractions become slower. Muscular fatigue is characterized by a longer latent period of muscular excitation and reduced excitability of the muscles involved. Excessive frequent contractions produce rapid fatigue. They take place when there is more load of work and when the capacity to work is exhausted. The result is the pain. In the case of workload, if the position of sitting and postures are changed in between the work, it will help muscles to retain some strength. *Hence the workload and rhythm of movement make an impact on the working capacity of the person doing some physical work* and consequently the amount of work done.

To some extent muscle fatigue is responsible for neck pain. A decrease in the working capacity of muscles has proportional relation with neural and chemical factors. Initially the fatigue is produced in the nervous centers, which actually master or regulate muscular work. The next place of the fatigue is the endings of nerves in muscle fibres. After this process, the character of the impulses reaching the muscles from the nervous system gets changed. The result is the decrease in the strength and speed of muscular contractions.

The speed with which the fatigue occurs depends upon the state of nervous system. State of nervous system can be made easy if the help of psychic and emotional factors is taken. This will increase the working capacity of the person.

Singing and music have been found very effective in increasing the working capacity and lowering the muscle fatigue. *If you are a good observer, you must have noticed that some good companies and even some banks (Some personalized branches of State Bank of India) have installed music channels over speakers so that their employees and the visitors get a soothing atmosphere free of tensions.*

As a matter of fact, the working capacity of the muscles depends upon the functional state of many systems of organs, cardiovascular, respiratory, endocrine etc. To reduce the muscle fatigue and increase the working capacity, a systematic training or physical exercise plays an important role.

Physical training brings about the changes not only in the muscles but also in all the other systems of organs like strengthening of cardiovascular and respiratory systems. All this type of exercise will improve the health and increase endurance besides development of the brain.

The finest example of adopting this procedure of physical exercise can be witnessed in big multinational companies now operating in India. Some of them have introduced essential physical exercise or Yoga for their workers and that too during the working hours of the company.

CHAPTER 4

CAUSES, SYMPTOMS AND GENERAL TREATMENT INCLUDING EXERCISES AND YOGA

CAUSES OF PAIN IN NECK

IF YOU ASK me frankly, I have not been able to find out the exact cause of the neck pains in different persons. This is my experience that persons with long neck are more prone to neck pains than persons with short necks. Both sexes get this attack but men are more in number to suffer from cervical spondylosis, probably because of their occupational activities. Their professional bindings to work at a place longer than the usual or prolonging the wrong postures in which they sit could be the cause. The people who travel on scooters, cars or jeeps on rough roads for a longer time in their professional binding (medical representatives, journalists, salesmen and executives etc.) are prone to this disease of neck.

Let us value the reasons of neck pain.

- The degenerative changes in the spine.

- Accident or traumas.

- Holding the head in one particular position over a long period as in the case of viewing cinema movie or driving a vehicle.

- Faulty postures in sitting, reading, writing or doing some work on computers.

- Mental stress and worries.

- Sleeping while resting the head on highly elevated pillows.

- Muscle fatigue and loss of working capacity.

SYMPTOMS

The start of cervical spondylosis is sudden and rapid but it never comes without prior warning. The person might have been experiencing uneasiness and slight pain in the past. Previous occasional attacks of stiffness of neck might have been there before the onset of cervical spondylosis. Such a pain can be in the form of stiffness of the neck and a little pressure of fingers on the neck cause pain. The pain can radiate towards the territory of the nerve on the shoulder girdle along the arm to the fingers. In the second instance of the pain attack, there may be tingling and numbness in the hand and occasionally giddiness and headache at the occipital area (back of head). The pain is of such a type that person affected may not get a wink of sleep during the night. The best part of this pain is that the severity of pain subsides after a few days but mild pain may continue for several weeks.

As a matter of fact, I have seen people not consulting the doctors for a mild nature of pain. The pain occurs but not so severe. The disease may progress into chronic stage. So far as the pain in the neck is concerned it becomes milder with the age.

(I have a patient who suffers from the neck pain while at work on the computer. He is working in a Bank. He never bothered to tell me about his ailment and pain till satisfied about the system of medicine i.e. Homoeopathy. He was not sure whether Homoeopathy could delete his sufferings. He initially came with his wife and children to have consultation for treatment of their minor ailments. After the treatment was done, his wife revealed about the neck pain of her husband. He had consulted many doctors and was used to take pain-killing medicines, frequently almost every day. During interrogation, his wife told that he is in the habit of taking more than 25 to 30 glasses of water each day. In the bank also, his peon was fed up to give him water every now and then. Seeing other symptoms, he was given *Bryonia*, 1M month back and till now he has not complained of the pain except few mild attacks now and then. He is not taking any pain-killer tablets now. The treatment is supposed to go on for some time so that further attacks, if any, could be monitored.)

STRESS - A CAUSE

In ancient India when the saints and yogis had a greater impact on the society, religion-wise and health-wise; the emphasis was that one should get rid of worldly stresses. It is a fact that body is governed by the physical, emotional, mental and spiritual powers working together to maintain a balance. Each of these aspects need mental and spiritual nourishment besides the physical uplink. Let us see an example as to how stress makes the condition of physical sickness more intensive.

When a man is hurt and his leg is broken, he is on the bed and cannot walk. His leg is plastered and he is on daily intake of medicines. So this injury has limited the freedom of the man to walk. A depression enters his mind and he is unable to interact with others on mental level because his physical contacts are no more. Because of his loneliness, he is mentally exhausted and this affects his ability to concentrate and make decisions. Till the injury is healed and he is able to walk, he is continuously under tension or stress. His injury will take more time to get healed because of the stress. Similarly if your boss in the office is aggressive to staff, there is a stressful environment created for employees, who in turn may get physical pains in head, neck and even indigestion. Those who are under stress are more prone to cervical spondylosis.

Today curative power of meditation has been recognized to ward off stress, and in turn the neck pain.

National Institute of Mental Health and Neuro-sciences, Bangalore has found that regular practice of Sudarshan Kriya Yoga (a technique of breathing exercises in Yoga) reduces the symptoms of mental depression. Sri Sri Ravi Shankar, founder of the Art of Liv-

ing Foundation at Bangalore, has promoted this technique. Researchers at All India Medical Institute of Medical Sciences are also working on this theory along with Pranayam, the traditional yogic breathing exercise. The method of Pranayam has been detailed in subsequent pages.

The best way to cope up with stress is to understand it. One has to learn the symptoms of being over-stressed. At different times of our lives, we react differently to similar stress. For example, working in the office is a routine and obviously a boss will always be there to monitor you. His duty is to guide you and your duty is to follow his advice. Where is the conflict? This has to be understood. If this sort of stress is understood, there will be no stress emotionally and in turn pain physically. The body shows the early signs of stress.

One must remember that he or she is an important person in his or her own life. If he or she has some pain, it is he or she who can tell where the pain lies. No doctor can find out where the pain is located. It is you who feel it and tell it. You need to look after yourself to be a healthy person.

TREATMENT IN GENERAL

At the start of disease, when the pain in the neck is sudden, it is better to take some rest for a short period till the severe pain subsides. If it does not go even after taking rest, it is befitting to wear a collar. We shall discuss about wearing a collar later when we discuss about physiotherapy treatment separately. **The collar is to give better rest to the strained or damaged muscles.** In this fashion, inflammation, if any, shall subside and pain will be abolished. Of course regular exercise of the neck helps. This will be discussed later. *It may be of importance to know that in the case of pain in the neck, it is advised that traction should not be applied to relieve pressure on the vertebrae.*

REST, THE FIRST REQUIREMENT

This is the best treatment when the pain is of new nature and is sudden after strains. You must have observed that in sport, the athletes running in a race are so much tired after reaching the finish line that they are forced to take rest to control their breathing. The same is true for a fatigued neck. After so much of stress on the computer or after a wrong posture of sitting/ sleeping, the neck needs rest. Rest is nothing but immobiliza-tion of the affected part. This helps the reduction of inflamma-tion or swelling, if any, and helps in abolishing the deformity due to muscle pulling and stretching.

One should also remember that doctors at the first instance advise rest and patients completely follow the instructions but *take excessive rest*. The patient must enquire from the doctor about the number of days the rest is to be taken. The thumb rule is that the rest to the neck should be given till the pain subsides. Rest means immobilizing the neck for few hours, pref-erably lying down without a pillow or resting the head on a thin pillow. Excessive rest is harmful because of the fact that keeping neck inactive for a longer period can result into atrophy of the muscles and total rigidity of the muscles. The rest to the neck should be systematic. By systematic, the purpose is to rest the whole of neck and the body. This will be helpful to reduce the inflammation, if any, but give comfort to the stretched muscles.

Rest effectively controls the disease process and is an effective method to avoid crippling of the patient and enable the patient to resume his daily chores.

HEAT THERAPY

Heat in some form is bound to give some relief in the case of stiff neck eliminating pain and soreness. This application of heat is more beneficial if it is done before taking up exercise of the neck. There are many types of heat-gadgets available in the market of which important are *electric heat pads and blankets, short-wave diathermy, hydro collator, hot water bottles, steam packs, many types of heat lamps, special tubs for baths and even hot air blowers.*

Electric heat pads and hot water bottles are more convenient. In case of acute stiffness and pain, the hot water bottle may be rested against the neck but not more than 10 to 15 minutes at a time.

One can use **hot packs** made out of folded soft cotton or woolen cloth. This pad can be easily made at home by folding a piece of cotton or woolen cloth (six to eight times folding) and then placing the same on the hot plate (Tawa in Hindi) to absorb heat. Now this cloth can be placed against the neck. After some heat application, the cloth will again be required to be heated. After the heat application, the neck is not to be exposed to cold air and it is better to wrap the neck.

In case, there is no inflammation or redness on the neck, **hot compress** can also be used.

Hot compress can be made out of a woolen cloth having

NECK EXERCISES

Turn Head to Left

Turn Head to Right

sufficient length to enable its wrapping around the neck. This cloth after folding is to be soaked in very hot water. The water should be wrung out completely and then wrapped around the neck. Important is that the patient should not go out of home in cold air after the compress and it would be better if the neck is covered by a thick cloth. The compress should be given 15 to 20 minutes everyday at least twice or thrice depending upon the severity of pain and stiffness of neck.

An infrared lamp is also an effective tool to apply heat. One thing should be kept in mind that the heat lamp is to be kept away from the skin at a distance of more than 45 cms or more and the duration of heat application should not exceed twenty minutes at a time. Here again, the neck should not be exposed to cold air and be properly covered.

EXERCISE OF NECK

If the learned readers of this book have my book, Know and Solve Thyroid Problems', they must be remembering the number of exercises I have suggested for controlling thyroid problems. Those who have not read, the same are produced here although with certain changes. Even if those exercises are repeated in the case of neck pains, they are helpful.

PURPOSE OF EXERCISE

It has been a traditional ordeal for the people in general to advise and conduct exercises as and when one feels lack of body strength or when someone gets cured of ailments by medicines

NECK EXERCISES

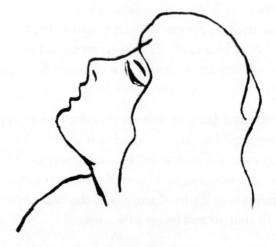

Backward Bending of Head

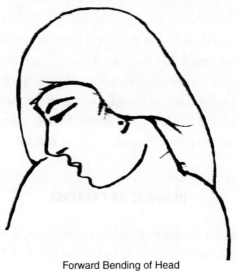

Forward Bending of Head

and doctors advise nutritional food with exercise and morning/ evening walk.

The *first purpose* of the exercise is that it strengthens the muscles that have been weakened by some disease or disorders. The *second purpose* of the exercise is that it will not allow the weakened muscles to get atrophied due to their non use or immobilization. The *third purpose* of exercise is that a routine adherence to regular exercise will help the neck and body joints to retain and regain the normal functions. It will not permit to get the neck stiff or reach a state of deformity due to immobility. Daily program of exercises should be carefully planned with the help of a therapist so that a correct method of exercise is followed and no deformity should take place.

NECK MOVEMENTS, THE BASIC EXERCISE

We have discussed about exercise of body and learnt that the purpose of exercise is also to allow adequate mobility and avoid jamming. In this connection, our subject allows sufficient margin for considering exercise of neck. Movement of neck is the prime theme to follow. Let us examine this aspect.

FORWARD AND BACKWARD MOVEMENT OF NECK

There is a special need for making the neck more flexible. For this, neck movement is essentially needed. The exercise is very simple and can be done while lying down on the bed. Place a lean pillow below the neck, not beneath the head. Now move the head forward and backward alternatively. If this exercise is done while standing, there will be more fatigue. If no fatigue is

NECK EXERCISES

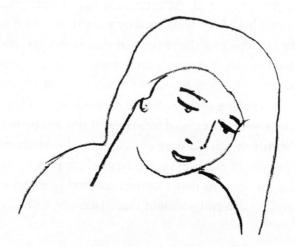

Head Left Side Bending on Shoulder

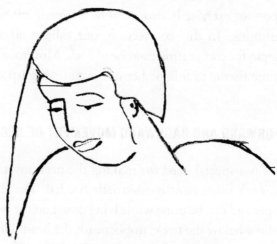

Head Right Side Bending on Shoulder

felt, this can be done in standing posture too. Start this exercise slowly and move the head ten times each side in the beginning. Later this can be increased to thirty times. *Please note that the movements in all the following exercises and above exercise should be very slow and no jerks are allowed while moving.*

SIDEWAYS MOVEMENT OF NECK

Now move the head sideways, stretching it as much as possible towards the right shoulder and then towards the left shoulder alternatively. The number of times this movement is made is already written above.

CIRCULAR MOVEMENT OF NECK

Sit down if you are performing the above exercises in lying position. Move the neck in a circle, first from left towards right side (anticlockwise) and then from right towards left side in a circular motion. It should be done very slowly. The number of times this movement should be done is mentioned above.

SPECIAL STRETCHING OF NECK

Apply some mustard oil or water on your right palm first. Now press it close to the left side muscles of neck and stretch it to left side as far as it can go. Again do the same thing with your left palm and stretch towards right side. Repeat the exercises for at least ten times everyday if not more.

NECK EXERCISES

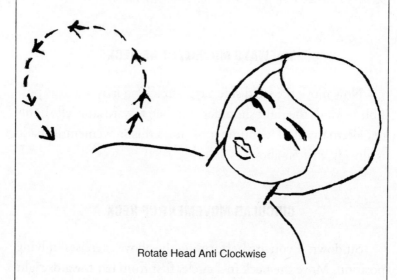

Rotate Head Anti Clockwise

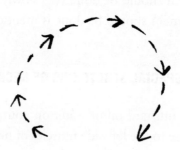

Rotate Head Clockwise

MASSAGE OF NECK

Lubricate your palms with mustard oil and give a massage to your neck glands in a slow motion. First massage the neck muscles below the chin with hollow of your palms in upward direction, say for ten to fifteen times. Now massage the neck from left to right and then from right to left. Next massage the muscles of the neck from the back -side, left to right and then from right to left.

NODS OF HEAD-HALF ASSENT AND FULL NEGATION FASHION

This is a type of exercise, has got very useful effect for those who work on computers and for those persons who feel vertigo sometimes. It has been tried on many patients and found very effective practically. This exercise can be done while at work in between the spells of long working routine on the computers.

Its practicing is simple. When someone agrees to opinion of others, he or she nods the head in affirmative. In the same manner, give a half nod to the head and then make a movement of neck sidewise as if denoting a complete negation of the opinion told. **This means a half yes and complete no (' Thodi haan, puri na' in Hindi, not in words but by nodding the head).**

FLYING THE NECK

Flying the neck means keeping the neck in the air for some time.

For this exercise, one has to lie on the stomach with his or her face down. Place a small pillow beneath the stomach and stretch the arms to the sides of hips keeping the palms upwards to the sky.

Now raise the upper body slightly while exhaling (breathing out). Hold the breath for four to five seconds.

Return to the starting position i.e. upper body back to the floor.

Repeat this exercise for five times and after two to three days of doing the exercise, increase the number of times to ten every day.

This exercise has been found very useful for salesmen and ladies in particular being of very simple nature. In recent cases when the pain in the neck has just started, this exercise is quite beneficial.

EXERCISE FOR BRACHIAL PAINS

This exercise is most suitable for the persons having neck pain associated with pains radiating to the arms and hands. This is also suitable for those patients who have long necks.

Take a chair with back and arm-rests (arm-chair). Now sit on this chair in such a fashion that your hands are resting on the arms of the chair and your back is not touching the back of chair. Sit erect and put all your body weight on your elbows and forearms keeping your hands-fingers on your stomach. Note that whole of your body weight is on the elbows and forearms and your feet are not supporting your weight. Your toes are touching the floor and not whole of soles. Sit in this posture for about ten to twelve minutes. If someone sees you in this posture, he will find you in a state as if your neck has gone inside your body and the shoulders are raised towards neck. This exercise should be done before going to bed every night and besides giving relief to your pains, it would induce good sleep as well.

STRESS MANAGEMENT

Allen Elkin, Director of Stress Management Center in New York has following to say to manage stress of continuous work. Conduct following act every half an hour of continuous work:

"Inhale deeply and hold your breath. At the same time, squeeze your forefingers and thumb together. Then, exhale slowly and completely. Release the tension in your fingers and let your jaw go slack. Breath deeply and slowly for several seconds." (Courtesy-Medical News-Woman's Era-December, 2002 issue)

This exercise is found useful for persons who work on computers. (For further guidance for computer operators, please see later in this book)

HEIGHT MEASUREMENT AND EXERCISE IN SPONDYLITIS PATIENTS

Height has a definite relation with the disease under reference especially when one develops a protrusion below the cervical area. A person suffering from cervical spondylitis or rheumatoid arthritis should measure his height once a month to find out the tendency in such a person to bend forward to relieve the pain in the neck. If some reduction of height is found after a few months on account of development of a hunch-back (Kyphosis) mostly found in ladies than men, there is need to correct the same by conducting a set of exercises as follows.

Stand erect against a wall in erect position and place your heels, buttocks, waist, shoulders and back of your head touching the wall. Now raise your hands above the head and stretch them upwards as far as they can reach. Do it for a few seconds and then return to normal position keeping your heels still with the wall. Do this act twice or thrice in a day whenever you get time. If you cannot raise your hands, just stand in the posture explained for some minutes, a number of times.

This type of exercise with hands raised upwards also increases height and children with short height should be encouraged to do it instead that they are told to hang on hands.

The patients who have a tendency of kyposis should also practice 'Pranayam', the act of holding breath and releasing. Here it is explained for the benefit of readers.

VIEWS OF VIDYAMARTAND
DR. SATYAVRATA SIDDHANTALANKAR
ON CERVICAL SPONDYLITIS

Dr. Siddhantalankar was a learned scholar of both Ayurveda and Homoeopathy and had written many valuable books on Homoeopathy. He was Member of Parliament and Vice Chancellor of Gurukul Kangri University also. In his most useful book "From Old Age to Youth through Yoga", he wrote about cure of cervical spondylitis through Yoga. He writes:

"Sometimes vertebras of the neck get jammed up after their ossification with the result that either the neck cannot bend or it cannot be kept erect. Sometimes there is a slip disc in which vertebras get jammed with the sensory nerves or there is inflammation of a vertebra, called spondylitis in which there is a swelling in the vertebras resulting in pain in all these cases. Exercises of the spinal column can prevent these mishaps, ***but all these exercises would be more harm than good when the spinal chord is affected by any of the three diseases- ossification, slip disc or spondylitis. These exercises should be taken as a preventive step, when the above complaints have not set in.**

To exercise the spinal column, stand erect with hands upwards, the arms closely touching the temples, and then bend forward making an effort to touch with fingers of the palms touching the right and left toes. Even if it is not possible.to reach the toes, bending in arch itself is good for spine. In the same position, one should bend backward trying to reach one's fingers towards the earth or one's heels as far as possible. Even if one cannot touch the earth or one's heels in bending backwards, one should try to bend backwards as far as possible. This will activate the spinal column and even in old age one would be able to stand and walk erect.

Do this bending - forward and backward - five times each.

---

* Bold letter is my incorporation because of the fact that it is very important. When either of these three diseases are there and the problem has become chronic, it is better not to conduct these exercises without the advise of the doctor. Regarding other neck exercises mentioned above, these might be done to prevent as well as cure acute cases of cervical spondylosis. It may also be noted that Dr. Siddhantalankar gave this quoting in reference with his subject of the book and not particularly for spondylitis.

PRANAYAMA

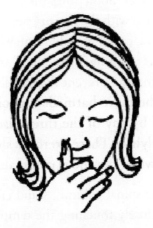

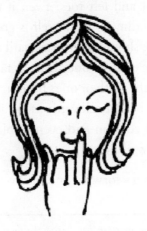

Expand the chest fully and uniformly, without allowing
the abdominal wall to bulge.

This bending involves contraction and relaxation and is helpful in preventing the jamming up of rigidity of the vertebras. It also keeps the sensory and motor nerves, passing through the spinal cord, healthy. These exercises are six in number - forward and backward, two slantwise, two in circles.

I Bend your body backward only as far as it can conveniently go and stay in this position till you finish the counting up to 300. Also give jerks and jolts to the body in this position, which helps in keeping the spinal column straight. Our back grows bent up in old age because most of our works are done in a forward bend-state of the body. To undo this reverse position should be maintained for a considerable time during exercise."

STRESS RELIVING YOGASANS HELPFUL FOR NECK PAIN

PRANAYAMA

The initial manifestation of life in a newborn baby is to take a deep breath. This first breathing is called *Prana* because without it the baby cannot survive. This ritual is without any training to the baby who takes breathing inside, retain it for a while and release the breathing. This is the process of breathing against which life commences. The life ends when this breathing ceases to exist. One can live without food or water for sometime but one cannot live without breathing. To attain good health, breathing has to be controlled and vitalized by some method of breathing in and breathing out. *Pranayama* is developed to look into this very aspect.

SHAVASANA

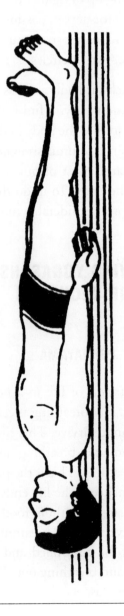

Lie down like a corpse. This asana relaxes the muscles and through them the mind, releasing tensions. Prescribed in hypertension.

Our ancient books on health reveal that there are three steps in conducting Pranayama. Inhaling air into the lungs with all one's strength is the first step called *Poorak*.

Holding back the air in the lungs is the second step called *Kumbhak*. Final exhaling the air from lungs is the third step called *Rechak*.

Poorak should be for about 10 seconds, Kumbhak should be for about 40 seconds and Rechak should be for 20 seconds. Actually this depends upon the capacity of the individual and is variable.

The pranayama suitable for neck and thyroid gland is that you inhale through left nostril and exhale through right nostril, using thumb and middle finger to close and open alternate nostril by pressing side of the nose. Do it for at least ten times. Now comes the second step. Inhale through left nostril and hold your breath for some time. Now release the breath i.e. exhale till the time you can do so and hold it for some time. This requires practice. The time you can hold should be your capacity to do so and in no case any longer time should be given beyond your capacity. This exercise creates a cooling effect in the body and increases the energy especially for women. After this exercise for a few days, you will find yourself a new person free of depression and tension. *It is my sincere advice to the readers that Yoga should not be done without proper training otherwise there may be some adverse effects.*

**SHAVASAN (CORPSE POSE)

Lie flat on your back on the floor and spread your feet keeping them at a distance of about two feet. Place a small pillow or folded blanket behind your head. Do not use a thick pillow. Your hands should be close to your body, touching the body. The palms should face upwards and hands should not be clenched. Close your eyes. Now feel relaxed and let your body be released or let loose. Try to feel the different parts of your body in contact with the floor.

For doing this, close your eyes and imagine your entire body, part by part is in touch with ground and is getting heavy. Do not get worried over this when you actually feel the limbs heavy. Throughout the practice of this asana, the worries and problems may keep appearing. Convince and tell yourself that these problems will receive your attention after a few minutes and that you are now practicing shavasana. Gently and slowly you will gain confidence and you will feel relaxed in all respects. During the whole of asana, feel free and relaxed as if you are dead so far as your body is concerned. Remain in this 'shav' or corpse position for some time, say at least ten minutes without any movement. While you are acting like a corpse, breathe deeply and take long breaths.

** Shavasan is one of the best asana for relief in stress. Dr. Datey, a renowned Heart Specialist of Bombay and recipient of Dhanvantri Award appreciate shavasan for releasing tensions. Explaining as to what happens when there is stress, he says, "There is at once an impulsive reaction. Stress is communicated to the brain by the five senses. *Thalamus* further transmits the impulse through the autonomous nervous system. Impulses are modified through *Shavasa*n. The shavasan is the best form of relaxation; it helps you even to change your nervous system. You would not react to a crisis as an average person would. The shavasan was once given to 47 patients with hypertension of various etiologies. A significant response was obtained in about 52 percent of the patients." (From book 'Old Age to Youth through Yoga' by Dr. Siddhantalankar)

PADMASANA

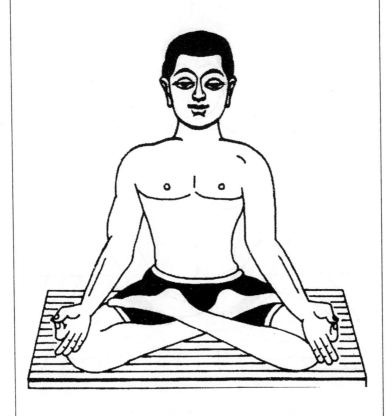

SIDDHASANA

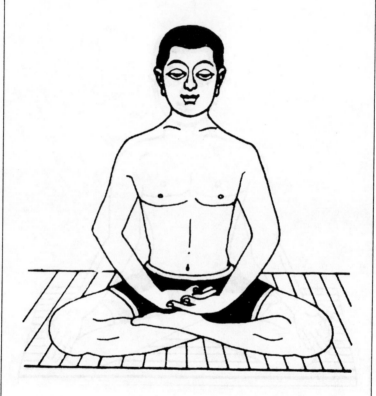

Sit with the left heel set against the perineum and the
right heel on the left one.

SARVANGASAN (STAND ON SHOULDERS)

Although there is a name given to this, stand on shoulders asana but I am particularly mentioning the easy way so that people can understand the posture. It influences the whole body and its functions, the entire human organism. This asana gives exercise to the neck. In this posture, you have to lie down on the floor and then raise your both legs upwards towards sky with the help of both your hands in such a position that the hands are pressed on the back (above hips) and elbows/forearm rest on the floor. The body and the neck will make a ninety-degree angle in this pose. The chin will be touching the chest. Keep your eyes stuck to both thumbs of your feet. Hold this posture for some time according to your capacity and bring back the legs to the ground very slowly without any jerks. The time of this posture can be increased according to the advice of your master. As I told you earlier, there is always a need for a master to learn this art.

PADMASAN AND SIDHASAN

After getting up early in the morning preferably before the sunrise, finish your daily routine of toilet and cleaning teeth etc. Now select a peaceful site where there is plenty of open air. Spread a clean mat over which you should take your seat. Fold your legs either in lotus asana (Padmasan) or Yoga mudra (Sidhasan). Lotus asana can be learnt from a person knowing Yoga. For this, you have to fold your left leg first onto your right thigh. Now fold your right leg over it. Or you can do the vice versa i.e. placing first right leg over the thighs and then the left leg over it. The heels will be beneath the navel region and the knees will be touching the earth. The soles of both the feet will be facing towards sky. Keep your back in a straight posture and spread your hands on your knees. Now fold thumb and index finger of both the hands together leaving the rest three fingers of each hand spread on the knee. This asana is a little difficult but in due course of practice, it can be done with ease. If this is found a little difficult, you can try yoga mudra. For attaining yoga mudra (Sidhasan), place your left leg-heel beneath right thigh so that the heel touches the middle area of anus and genitals. Now put your right leg over it in such a fashion that the sole of right foot faces sky. Now place your hands on your lap, on the heel of the right leg. The hands are to be kept one above the other facing sky. Please note that the heels of the legs should not be kept over the genitals. This is much easier asana and can be a starter for doing your 'pranayama'. Pranayama is the process of breathing smoothly, inhaling and exhaling from the nostrils as per the prescribed procedure.

Note: All these Asana should be done in consultation with a Yoga teacher who should be told about the neck problems. Although these asana are not directly related with neck problems but surely these would fetch best results body is considered one unit and neck is no separate organ from Body. Once stress of life is eliminated, all the medicines will work wonders.

Important: It is also to be noted that any exercise, which aggravates pain during or after the exercise should not be done and guidance from a physiotherapist becomes essential in such case. Exercise should be done in a slow and gradual fashion so that the spinal ligaments may get a chance to achieve their natural elasticity and not damaged due to additional and sudden force so applied by rigorous exercises. Some people have an illusionary opinion that initial pain in the neck, when in the act of starting neck exercises on the very first day, is due to direct attack on the paining spot and the pain will be gone after exercises are continued for more than two or three days. Generally this does not happen and the pain will go on increasing.

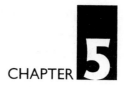

CHAPTER **5**

PROPER POSITIONS AND POSTURES

THE AMAZING ERECT POSTURE

H UMAN BODY is a wonderful creation of Almighty and differs very much from animals in one major aspect that it stands on two feet. It has a majestic erect position or posture, which is offered by our spine. Our spinal curves are made in such a fashion that they allow flexibility to the maximum provided these curves are not misused by adopting wrong postures. In the fourth week of pregnancy, the spine and the nervous system start to form in the embryo. In the seventh week, there are small spinal movements. In twelve to fourteen months, nearly all the organs including spine are formed. The spinal curves are absent at the birth of a baby and during the first few weeks of life it is a continuous curve when the baby is in the womb. The basic curve develops when the baby tries to raise his head, tries to sit, tries to crawl, stand walk and run in consequent progressive fashion. Once the spinal curves are formed, it becomes obvious that the child should stand erect. This posture of standing erect is the normal state of human body and it should be maintained throughout life. It is this posture that the army and police officials give utmost importance. The first command to the armed forces to the Jawans is 'attention' upon which the solider is supposed to stand erect. The second command is generally 'stand at ease', which is also to stand erect but with leisurely spread legs and hands behind position. To stand erect is in both the postures. This shows that standing erect is a must for an army person. In other words, to keep alert and fit, standing erect is a blessed slogan for keeping good health.

THE SURPRISING FLEXIBILITY OF SPINE AND NECK

You must have observed village lasses carrying pitchers full of water, one upon the other, and they walk a very long distance to fetch water. Just observe their gait. It is so graceful to watch them carrying a load and balancing them too. It is all an example of how spine can perform miracles. The head, neck and the spine are burdened with load of water and pitchers and yet the spine works as a shock absorber to bear the burden and still walk erect. The balancing act of circus players is also another example. Their feats are full of amazing twisting of spine consisting of surprising flexibility. See another example. In

Maharashtra during Lord Ganesha Utsav or festival, young boys of the streets perform a unique balancing act of making human pyramids by standing one upon the other to reach the top and break the hanging pitcher. The spine has a tremendous capability of flexibility and so is the neck. If it is mobile, there is no reason why neck pain or spinal pains should occur.

CORRECT POSTURES FOR AVOIDING NECK PAIN

In view of the above explanations, it is very important that the posture of sitting, standing and walking should be correct so that there is no extra burden on the neck. A wrong and even slightly defective posture when continued for a longer time can result in strains on the joints and bring about pains. Those who already suffer from neck pain, can invite insidious attack of arthritis or aggravate the existing disease. A careful self-examination of one's posture of work can be done from time and time and rectified. I have seen the parents hinting at children to sit straight without stooping. This is a good practice and the children should be guided. We have already detailed about some exercises for neck, which will certainly help obtain correct postures. The first thing to learn and to guide the children from the very young age is to make them alert through correct postures. How to carry the weight of the body is the first lesson, a child should be taught.

There should not be any hump in the back when the child learns to sit, stand and walk.

It stands true for adults also but the training should be from the childhood otherwise correct manner of walking would be little difficult. If the back has a hump or in other words, if the head is let loose to hang over the body and not kept erect, the vertebrae get contracted and neck sunk down in the chest. This is a major reason for neck pain, headaches and pain in the arms. There should be balanced weight and pressure on both the legs. If someone is putting extra pressure on one leg while walking or standing, there will be extra strain on the pelvis and lumbar spine besides that the muscles become tense. *Equal distribution of body weight on the legs is a must to avoid backaches and neck pains.*

When we sit, stand, walk or drive a vehicle there should not be any bending of spine, there should not be any stooping. Some people have the habit of sitting on the scooter or bike seat with bent back. While their hands are straight on the handle of the bike in a straight manner, the mind is alert and watchful on the road and is totally engaged on careful driving, the back is totally forgotten. It is a common tendency and one cannot remember to keep the back erect. Such people with bent back while driving bikes are more prone to body aches than those who drive with erect posture. Similar is true for car drivers. First of all the seat of the car should be adjusted nearer to the steering wheel and if still there is margin for the back having a space between it and the back of seat, a small pillow should be placed. Now a days, this problem of space between back and back of driving seat is somewhat less because the latest rules of driving have made wearing of a seat-belt compulsory. It is a very useful move for health of back and neck.

Erect and only erect is the correct method to sit, stand, walk or drive a vehicle.

The sad thing about all these matters explained above is that we are not much conscious about these basic guidelines and doctors of the orthodox system of medicines also do not bother much to tell the parents of the children in a very precise manner. In the olden days, when I was studying in the primary school in Amritsar, I remember one particular teacher very conscious about the way we the boys of the class sit. If someone from us were found sitting in a bent posture, he would come and hit the back with a wooden rule. This type of teaching is not seen now a day when beating of the school children is thought to be an offense.

Both parents and teachers should be watchful of the children's posture of sitting, if not standing or walking. The very sitting posture of the child, while he or she reads/studies can be corrected by frequent reminding the child of his or her bad posture.

HOW TO STAND AND SIT ERECT

Not standing or sitting erect causes all the aches and pains in the cervical, dorsal and lumbar regions of the spine. If we study our biological background, we shall find that cervical and lumbar curves have emerged after the man reached a stage of standing erect. Darwin's Theory of evolution says that the man walked on four and the erect position was attained after thousands of years. There was a gradual improvement in reaching our standing position from crawling on legs and hands. Once this was achieved, it became very useful for running and walking fast for the man. This sort of stage of standing was achieved only after standing erect. Such is the importance of standing erect. The curves in the spine make the man erect and when

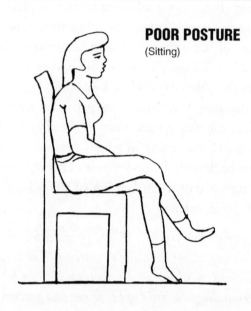

POOR POSTURE
(Sitting)

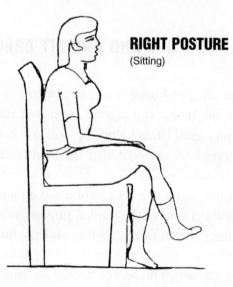

RIGHT POSTURE
(Sitting)

these curves are more than required, it becomes a causative factor for neck and back pain. The most vulnerable to such excessive curves in the spinal joints are internal derangements in fifth and sixth cervical and fourth and fifth lumbar vertebrae. These are the regions of spine where cervical and lumbar fatty accumulation is more significant. (Lordosis). If lordosis is allowed to go on, the subject is more prone to neck and back pains. This is why emphasis is always upon the child to see that he or she sits and stands in an erect position. Once this sort of guidance is imparted in the childhood, the future can be stored with relaxed feeling so far as these two ailments are concerned.

THE PLACE TO SLEEP, THE BED AND THE PILLOW

Both neck pain and back pain have a definite bearing with the type of bed, one is using. Guidance is needed to the people on the right choice of bed so that the spine and the body receive the rest required without any damage to the spine. People use different types of beds with different types of mattresses and cots. In the villages, wooden cots with wooden planks are most common. Cots having a woven coir string textured ('Baan' in Hindi) in the four frames of wood, wooden frame having a texture of cotton strip called 'Niwar' in Hindi are also used in villages and small towns where manuals are available for constructing and straightening the strings. Over these wooden planks, coir string net or cotton strip net, the cotton mattress is used in winter and cold seasons.

The times are changing now. With the hot wind blowing from city life to the rural life, the beds are changing and surely

STANDING POSTURES

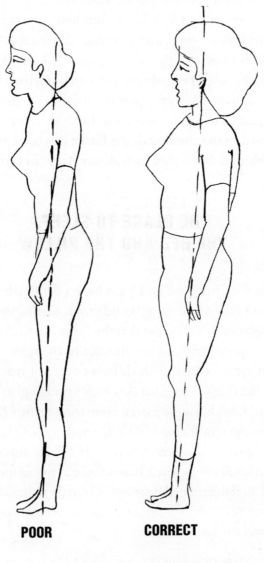

POOR   **CORRECT**

Differing Unequal Pressure on Joints - Spine - Neck

for the worst if the health point of view is main consideration. Following blindly the so-called luxurious living of the people of cities, the village and small town people are using foam mattresses instead of conventional cotton mattresses. Even if foam is avoided, cotton mattresses with springs beneath are also used. It has been made a status symbol and as dowry in the marriages, foam mattresses are given and demanded. The thicker the foam, the better is said to be the living standard of the bridal family. The idea behind this type of thick foam or springs is that the ideal bed is one, which has more of sinking power. As soon as one sits on this type of bed, he should sink into it and feel the jump. This is worst kind of bed for the spine. Many of those who suffer from backaches and neck pains are the people who sleep on these 'sinking' beds.

Why are these beds bad for body? Our body has three main dividers so far as the body weight is concerned. The head and neck are the lighter parts, the trunk or the part from neck to pelvis is the heaviest part and the hips and legs are heavier parts. When the body sinks into the foam mattress, the heaviest part of the body sinks deeper in the bed and the next lighter part is raised. This makes a wrong curvature of the spine and puts lot of unwanted strain on it. This is one part of the game of sleeping. The second part is still worse. It is using thick pillows. The weight of the head is less and it is raised on higher elevation than the body, the person feels more comforts when he uses thick pillow. The curve of cervical gets more flexibility when a thick pillow is used. This pose gives a lot of strain to the neck muscles as well. Our body has a wonderful capability of standing all the strains or wrong postures, if these are temporary but if someone goes on practicing these wrong postures of sleeping, the body will certainly cry or make you cry with pains. Pro-

STANDING POSTURES

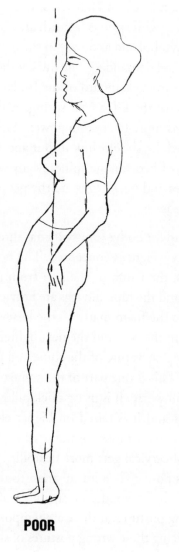

POOR   **POOR**

Differing Unequal Pressure on Joints - Spine - Neck

longed excesses of bad posture of spine on thick 'sink-in' beds weaken the ligaments, bring in minor changes or displacements in the intervertebral joints and finally break down the mechanism of body producing pains. In ancient India when students were required to get their primary education in 'Gurukuls', the students were told to sleep either on floor or wooden beds. This was the best bed to straighten the spine wherein the lumbar lordosis is best maintained due to structural peculiarity of the lumbar spine.

The very construction of the cervical and lumbar vertebrae is such that if one lies flat on the floor without a mattress, both the cervical and lumbar lardosis are in the posture of good relief. Why this sort of posture is beneficial can be also explained by the example of running on the sand. When one runs or even walks on the sand dunes, extra pressure is exerted on the spine due to cushioning of sands on the soles of feet. One has to exert more to make moves. In the same way, when mattress is in between the body and the floor, this is likely to hamper the curves of the spine. Those who suffer from cervical spondylosis, this posture should be maintained for some days. *The best method to do this is to lie on the floor for some time after the day's hard work and tiredness.* This will relax the muscles and the spine. In the starting of the posture of sleeping on the floor, one may experience a little discomfort or slight pain in the back and cervical region but this will be over after some time.

"Sleeping on proper bed strengthens the muscles of heart and also it induces good sleep. One develops good patience and health also improves. Sleeping on wrong type of bed has an opposite effect. By sleeping on a wooden cot with tied strings help eliminate rheumatism and cough. He, who sleeps on bare

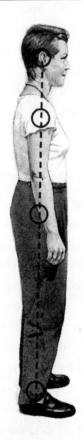

CHECK YOUR STANDING POSTURE

To improve your standing posture, follow these steps:
- Breathe deeply.
- Relax your shoulders, hips, and knees.
- Think of the ears, shoulders, hips, and ankles as a series of dots. Now, adjust your body to connect the dots in a straight line.
- Tuck your buttocks in just a bit if you need to.

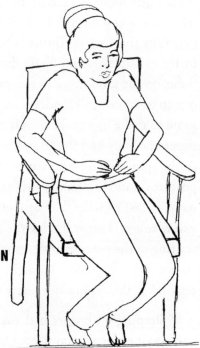

POSTURE TO RELIEVE PAIN IN BRACHIAL NEURALGIA

Sitting on armchair with body weight on elbows & forearms

earth will be more strong and virile. A wooden bed is 'vatal'. He, who sleeps on wooden plank will get cured of all his pains."

The above comment in inverted comma is the meaning of a Sanskrit Shaloka written in Book 'Bhav Parkash' by Shri Rajeshwer Dutt Shastri. (Courtesy: Book 'Cure' by Dr. Krishan Murari Modi). According to Ayurveda, all the aches and pain in the cervical region are due to 'Vata' or the air.

SLEEPING POSTURE

Sleeping postures also vary. Those who suffer from cervical spondylosis should try to sleep on the left or right side instead of continuous sleeping on the back. While sleeping on the sides of the body, one should lie with the legs slightly flexed or bent at the knees towards the abdomen. This will offer a greater sense of relaxation to the muscles.

THE TYPE OF BED RECOMMENDED IN CITIES

Those who already suffer from cervical spondylosis with frequent attacks should either lie on floor or hard wooden-ply bed with a mat (Durry in Hindi) beneath during summer. In winter, they can sleep on a hard wooden-ply bed with a mattress beneath. The mattress should have a thin layer of cotton sewed and tied in such a fashion that there is no sinking-in when sitting on it. The best way to ascertain such type of mattress is that while sleeping on it, the spine should feel straight. Such types

LEARNING SAFE BODY MECHANICS

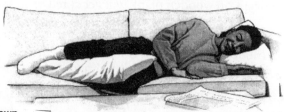

Lying Down
- When lying on your side, bend your knees and place a pillow between them.
- If you lie on your back, put a pillow under your knees.
- If you lie on your stomach, place a pillow under your abdominal muscles.

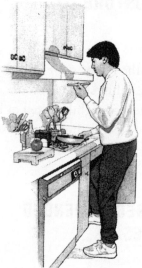

Standing
- Bend your knees slightly to take stress off your lower back.
- Wear shoes that support your feet. This helps keep your spine aligned.
- If you must stand for long periods, raise one foot slightly. Rest it on a low shelf or Shift feet often.

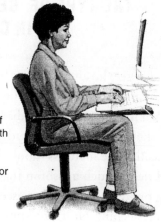

Sitting
- Sit in chairs that support your back. Keep your ears in line with your hips. If needed, support your lumbar curve with a rolled-up towel or lumbar roll.
- Your knees should be level with your hips. Your feet should be flat on the floor or on a footrest.

of mattresses are available in the market and can be made to order as well. Use of this type of **firm mattress** is only beneficial when it is placed on a hard bed or floor. A person suffering from rheumatic diathesis will have a benefit if he or she sleeps on a hard board bed overlaid by the above type of firm mattress. The best use of this type of mattress is to avoid use of pillows and if pillow avoiding is not possible, 'semal' cotton pillow can be used. Hard bed and no pillows is the best recommendation.

USE OF 'SEMAL' TYPE OF COTTON-PILLOWS

The pillow should contain *'Semal' type of cotton.* Semal in Hindi is the name of cotton type. This cotton is highly flexible and grows on big trees mostly found in Bihar, Bengal and Assam. It is easily available in all cities of India. As a matter of fact, pillows having *semal* cotton are readymade available in the market. Those who suffer from cervical spondylosis should preferably sleep on floors or hard wooden beds without pillows. Lying on one side of the body with arm extended beneath the head will give better relief to the neck pains. In case of discomfort felt without the pillow, one can use this 'semal' pillow initially. Gradually after a few days, the pillow can be removed.

MARRIAGE, DINNER AND DRINK PARTIES

In the modern era, gatherings in the form of cocktail and dinner parties have become the order of the day in both social and business life. One cannot avoid the same and if someone has cervical spondylosis problem, he/she has to keep in mind

LEARNING SAFE BODY MECHANICS

Bending and Lifting
- Bend at your knees and hips instead of your waist. Do your best to keep your hips in line with your shoulders.
- Hold objects close to your body to limit strain on your back.
- Lift your body and the load at the same time. Let your leg muscles do most of the lifting.

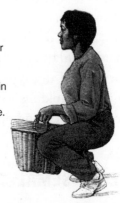

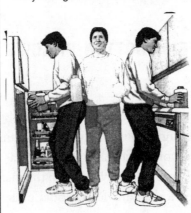

Turning
- Think of your upper body as one straight unit, from your shoulders at your buttocks.
- Turn with your feet, not your back or knees. Point your feet in the direction you want to go. Then step around and turn. Maintain your spine's three curves.

Reaching
- Store common items between shoulder and hip level.
- Get close to the item. Use a stool or special reaching tool, if you need to.
- Tighten your abdominal muscles to support your back. Use the muscles in your arms and legs (not your back) to lift the item.

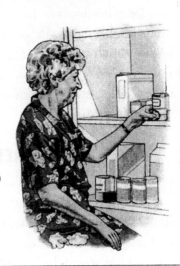

that food and drinks are not taken more than the minimum required to mix up with the people. Moderate drinking of liquor once in a week is not going to make any serious harm to the disease. The drinks should not be a cocktail or a mixture of variety of liquors but a single type of drink. If it is whisky, let it be whisky alone without even soda. Similarly do not overload your stomach with food. In most of the parities, the fashion is standing and taking the food or drink (Buffet). For spondylosis patients, it is not advised to take meals while standing for a long time at one place or continue moving about. It is better for the spine to sit down for a while. Take your meals and find out a chair to sit.

DRIVING A VEHICLE

If you are going for a long drive to a hill station or otherwise, it is better to take some rest after one hour of driving. Stop the car after every hour, get down from it, stretch your hands above, turn your neck side-wise for a while and walk about on the road for a minute or so. Now you are ready for further driving.

LIFTING OF LOAD

If you are going for marketing and collection of groceries or vegetables etc., it is suggested that the load of goods purchased be divided in two bags, packets or baskets. Each of the bags should have approximate equal amount of weight and you should carry one bag each in each hand. After walking for a while, it is

GOOD POSTURE FOR AVOIDING NECK PAIN

Sleeping on Hard Bed Without Pillow

better to place the load on the road, take some rest for about thirty seconds and then again carry the bags. In the event of one bag in your hand and the weight can be divided in two parts to carry in each hand, it is better to shift the bag from one hand to the other after walking for a while. If the load of bag is more than your lifting capacity, hire a laborer. If this is also not possible and you have to lift the bag yourself, better carry it in rucksack or in a bag evenly balanced between the shoulders.

At home, if a bucket full of water is to be carried by you, it is better to slide along the floor instead of lifting. If this sliding is not possible, make the bucket light by draining half of the contents. If some heavy load is required to be lifted from the floor in your home, do not bend the waist to lift it. You can squat and pick it up while keeping the back and neck straight. Bend your knees instead of back.

TYPE OF SHOES TO WEAR

Foot is an important part of our body and without it we cannot stand or move. The standing and moving has a great link with our brain, neck and shoulders. You must have observed that in south India, people are not accustomed of using any footwear at least in their houses. On roads, we cannot avoid using footwear but a caution is needed on this account. The shoes should be comfortable, when walking with, and should not develop much of heat. Leather shoes are supposed to be best for footwear. As a matter of fact, different kinds of activities like sports, mountaineering, and long walks require different kinds of shoes. In bath-rooms, one should wear 'chappal' having non-skidding sole.

Footwear is a very important factor in the preventive measures. *Shoes with high heels should not be used. Mostly ladies wear high-heeled sandals and these are not good for spine. The spine is thrown out of line by use of high-heeled shoes and pain in the neck or back is not avoidable.*

AVOID THE FOLLOWING POSTURES POSITIONS

- When you know the type of road you will be required to drive is rough and bumpy, avoid journey on scooter, motor-bike and jeeps. When the journey is by bus or truck and it is unavoidable, better to wear a high foam rubber or felt-collar on the neck to avoid jarring and jolting of neck. *The collar can be selected in consultation with the attending physician or the physiotherapist.*

- If you are planning to see a movie in a cinema hall, better not to see the movie when you had already had a attack of neck pain the other day. You will be required to sit in an awkward position for a long time of three hours watching the movie and this may bring on the pains.

- If you are having fits of coughs and sneezing, better take bed rest and treat the disease by appropriate medicines. Excessive coughing may aggravate the neck pains.

- Your daily chores should be adjusted in such a manner that there is least strain on the neck.

- Excessive exercise and fatigue should be avoided.

GUIDELINES FOR COMPUTER USERS

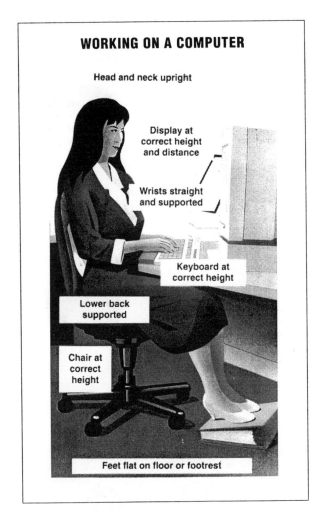

WORKING ON A COMPUTER

Head and neck upright

Display at correct height and distance

Wrists straight and supported

Keyboard at correct height

Lower back supported

Chair at correct height

Feet flat on floor or footrest

Those who use computers mostly complain about the stress and pain in the neck region. Here are a few guidelines for them.

- Use high table to avoid a stoop while working on the computer.

THINK BACK THROUGHOUT THE DAY

Warm Up for the Day
Do a few slow, catlike stretches before starting your day. This simple warm-up can soften your disks, stretch your back muscles, and help prevent injuries.

Shift Positions Often
At work and at home, change positions often. This helps keep your body from getting stiff. Stand up or lean back while you sit. If you can, get up and move every half-hour.

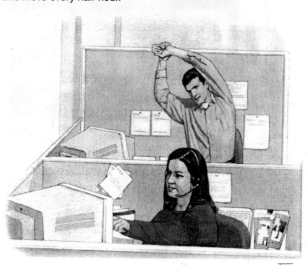

- Your eyes should be straight on the computer and the computer should be in alignment with the eyes.

- In typing on the board of computer, the height of the table should be so adjusted that you feel comfort on your spine and there is no bending at the lumbar region while typing.

- Use a chair with a firm seat without cushion while sitting. Keep your back straight giving full support to the hips and the back. Your feet should rest on something a little higher than the floor level. The use of low chairs having thick cushions should be avoided.

- Do not work on computer continuously for hours. Take a break in between, say after every half an hour. During this break, first thing to do is to keep your palms over the eyes in such a way that the palms do not touch the eyes and make a cup over the eyes with a gap between the eyes and palms. Cover your eyes in this fashion for a minute or so and you will find adequate relief in eyestrain.

- Now stretch your hands above your head and spread the fingers. Hold them for a while and lower the hands. Do this two to three times.

- To give rest to your tired hands due to typing, place the bottom of your right palm over the bottom of your left palm and press it for a while. Now repeat the same with the bottom of your left palm pressed by the bottom of your right palm.

- Keep your back straight on your chair and now look towards right shoulder moving your neck slowly. Keep this posture for a while and now repeat this with change of direction i.e. look towards your left shoulder moving the neck slowly. After doing this for two times on both sides, make your neck straight and nod slowly three times.

- Now lay your neck on the shoulder to left shoulder and then to right shoulder as if you are allowing your head to sleep on the shoulder. Do it three times both sides.

- Move your hips forward to the edge of the chair. Sit straight and keep your hands on the rest of chair. Now turn your body to right side as if you are looking behind. Remain in this posture for a while and now do it again turning your body to left side. Do it three times.

- Push your chin forward to stretch the jaw and neck.

- Sit straight on the chair. Roll each shoulder forward and around then back and around. Do it three times.

- Lift your each shoulder simultaneously up to your ear and bring it down. Do it three times.

(Please also see previous pages for exercise of neck, stress management).

CHAPTER 6

DIET SUGGESTIONS FOR CERVICAL SPONDYLOSIS

EARLIER IN this book, you have read about effect of stress on the body. Diet plays a role in removing stress, if it is adequate. When the body is in continuous stress of overwork, anxiety, insufficient diet, lack of sleep and lack of exercise, it is likely to be more prone to various diseases. It is the pituitary gland at the base of brain that starts the work of repairing damages in the body. (Read my book on Thyroid problems for detailed study of endocrine glands). The pituitary gland secretes hormones like ACTH and STH. These are taken to the two adrenal glands (situated above the kidneys) to utilize them. They stimulate various organs of the body to increase activities and repair the damaged cell of body. They draw Proteins from thymus and lymph glands, convert them into sugar and broaden the activities of liver, heart, kidneys and other organs. If the diet containing proteins, vitamins already exist in the body, the stress will be very less and there would not be more damage to the body cells. *Deficiency of the vitamins and proteins can limit the hormone production and cause a sort of degeneration of the adrenal cortex. So the nutrients are essential part of diet.*

We have already discussed about spur forming in the vertebral joints wherein the joints get cemented together, especially in spondylitis. Once this happens, nothing can be done but this is the view of many Allopaths, not Homoeopaths. The process of spur formation or cementing of joints can be reversed by diet planning and this diet should be given for a long time.

One must remember that a person, who is **regulated in diet** and recreation, restrained in action, disciplined in sleeping and walking, gets rid of all sorrows. Take simple and nourishing food and avoid chilies and aerated drinks. Never eat for enjoyment but eat for survival. (An old saying)

It is obvious that most of the patients come to Homoeopathy when they have already tried their hands at Allopathy and Ayurveda. Taking allopathy means, intake of Aspirin is a must in some form or the other to eliminate pains of neck. One should remember that Aspirin destroys huge quantity of vitamin C in the body. There is a need to give the body its requirement of vitamin C if the patient has taken Aspirin. See another case, if the patient has taken cortisone in some form during his medication, he will lack in vitamins B and C and have deficiency of proteins. They should not take much of salt. Let us have a view about the diet now - a diet which should be quite *nutrient in nature.

RECOMMENDED DIET

- Fresh *green and leafy vegetables* should be taken. Salad should be always included in the meals. Spinach, carrot and beet juices can also be taken.

- *Proteins* should be balanced in the diet. Milk is the best diet for getting proteins. Yogurt is also very good and it should be taken daily. This will act as antibody for the Aspirin consumed by the body in the past. Taking cereals, rice, and potatoes should be reduced and one should take brown bread instead of white bread. Brown bread is now easily available in the market.

- *Among fruits,* seasonal fruits are the best selections. Unstrained juices from oranges, grapes and pineapples are supposed to be good for rheumatic patients.

- On *cooking oils,* it is better if the oil taken by the regional people is adopted. For example, Punjab, UP, Rajasthan, Gujrat people mostly prefer to take either mustered oil or groundnut oil. Mustered oil is taken in west Bengal, Bihar, and Orissa and northeast states. Coconut oil is preferred in southern states. These are traditional oils being taken by the people in their respective states. Oils like sunflower, rapeseed, peanut, soyabean, corn etc. are recently introduced in the market and should be taken on the advise of doctors. All these oils may be used for cooking and light frying and *Ghee, butter oil or cream* should be used sparingly. Half to one teaspoon of ghee in a day used on Chapatti or in vegetable is not going to create any problem and is good for rheumatic diseases including cervical spondylosis. (A view)

- Use of *refined sugar* should be brought to minimum. The

body does require sugar and it can be met with by use of fruits, fruit juices, 'Gur', 'Shakar' and honey at times.

■ Processed, refined, canned or *tinned food-stuff* should not be taken.

■ If you are addicted to *tea taking,* reduce your requirement to two or three cups of tea a day and not more. The tea should not be strong and be diluted with milk.

■ One cup of milk should be taken at night, if not one glass full. Regarding *milk,* it is advised that whole cream milk should be taken from government Dairy but the milk should be taken after boiling and removing the cream out of it. By cream, I mean 'Malai' in Hindi. Milk should be taken as hot as the room temperature.

■ *With intake of homoeopathic medicines,* vitamin supplement is not going to harm the body. One can take vitamin B complex, vitamin C, vitamin D and vitamin E along with homoeopathic medicines depending upon the requirement if advised by the doctor.

■ If the disease has been categorized under rheumatism and *arthritis,* it is better to avoid cakes, biscuits, calcium foods in excess, meat, citrus fruit, white sugar, almonds, cashew nuts, coconuts, walnuts, peanuts and aerated waters.

■ *On alcohol,* it is not recommended for arthritis patients. We know that freshness is felt after a good sleep but after drinking excessive alcohol, there may be unconsciousness but never a feeling of freshness. The action of alcohol is on vital organs like brain, heart, kidneys and liver. The extent of effects of alcohol depends upon the concentration of alcohol in the blood and brain cells. Alcohol also causes inflammation of stomach and it should not be considered as a digestive tonic. Excessive use of alcohol should always be avoided. If someone thinks that the *pain in the neck gets less after drinking liquor, he or she is totally mistaken.*

■ *Non- vegetarian* food should always be avoided. Soft boiled eggs, fish and chicken can be taken by those who are strictly non-vegetarians.

■ The *quantity of food* intake should be about 10-20 percent less than the actual hunger, especially at dinner- time. If you are in the habit of taking three chapattis, take two at dinner-time.

■ On *water intake,* it is better not to take water with lunch and dinner. Take water one hour before or after the meals. A maximum quantity of water to be consumed in between meals is half a glass, if you cannot resist taking water. One can take plenty of water during day-time.

■ Finally, the food should be taken at regular intervals and one should *avoid strenuous work immediately after lunch and dinner.* One should not go in for cycling, taking bath and indulge in intercourse immediately after meals. The *sex* can be enjoyed only when one is relaxed and not when the body busy in digesting food. One should not go to sleep immediately after taking dinner. Some walk is essential before going to bed.

NUTRITION

What is exactly meant by nutrition? Let there be no confusion. Scientists on this special science have conducted a lot of research. In big hospitals, Dieticians are employed to help the doctors. The research shows that the body's development and optimum functioning of different tissues need at least 40 nutrients in the diet. These nutrients are in the form of fatty acid (one at least), vitamins (15 in all), and minerals (14). From these nutrients, the body synthesizes various enzymes, different hormones, co-enzymes and activators to make various organs healthy. A deficiency of any of these nutrients in the food consumed over a long period may lead to a condition of body-stress. This stress turns to body illness. (We have already read about stress and its relation with cervical spondylosis). During the period of disease, which is a form of stress, the requirement of the body for proteins, vitamins and minerals grow speedily. Of course this depends upon the severity of the case and it is at this juncture that generous supply of nutrients be made in the diet. This should also be ensured that nutrients given to the body, are digested by body and that they assimilate with or without use of medicines. This is the duty of doctor to take care when treating cases of cervical spondylosis.

USE OF EGGS

Many people have a misconceived idea that eggs are more nutritious and easily digestible. It is a myth only. The research on eggs has proved that 100 gram of eggs provide 160 calories. On the other hand, 100 gram of pulses, grain, peas etc. provide 330 to 370 calories. The oil seeds provide 450 to 550 calories, and groundnut/soyabean give 900 calories. Butter and pure ghee have highest calories and are supposed to be best for energy (90 calories). It is also believed that eggs are more nutritive and beneficial for the health of children and old persons. This is again a myth. Chemical analysis has proved that eggs have got much cholesterol, which is deposited in the liver and blood vessels. Taking fried eggs is more dangerous for digestion and health. Those who take too many eggs from childhood, they suffer from many liver, brain and kidney diseases in the later life. Excessive use of eggs can be the cause of gout, rheumatoid arthritis and constipation.

Those who think that eggs are good source of protein, will be astonished to find that eggs have 13.3 percent of protein whereas pulses have 24 percent of protein. Groundnut, soyabean and powdered milk have 31, 43 and 38 percent of protein respectively. Actually eggs are deficient in iron, calcium and magnesium. "They do not contain carbohydrates and their tendency is to favor putrefactive decomposition in the intestine rather than to encourage fermentative organism to develop", says Dr. E.V. McCallum, a great authority on newer knowledge of nutrition.

CHAPTER 7

FAQS ON NECK PAIN AND THEIR ANSWERS

Here are some basic questions a layman would like to have answers.

Q.1. What are the most common reasons for neck pain, and what can the average patient do to avoid any further damage?

Answer: The most common cause for neck pain is related to the disc located between the bones of the neck. Problems in the neck can also cause arm and neck pain. If the spinal cord is compressed, there may be pains all over the body. This is quite a serious condition, although it does not occur with high frequency. Most of the problems in the neck are due to a disc that may cause a neck pain further radiating to the arms, and possibly the hands. If the spinal cord is affected, the result will be difficulty in walking, problems in maintaining balance, hand-numbness, and sometimes problems with the legs. When the spinal cord is compressed, some doctors say that surgery is the best treatment. If the spinal cord is not compressed, medical treatment with conventional medicines or alternative therapy like Homoeopathy, Ayurveda and Physical therapy can be tried.

Q.2. If a person is having upper neck pain all the life due to working on computer or working on the desk with a wrong posture for a longer time, what can be done?

Answer: All the life means slight pain attacks in between the spells of continuous work and some rest to the neck. This is a common problem. Frequently people have occupational difficulties if their working place is not fitted with suitable type of chairs and tables and where height of both the chair and table is not ideal for work. It is necessary in such cases that the working tables, chairs and also the environment be examined to assure that both the back and neck positions are normal and comfortable during long hours of work on computers. By environment, I mean that one should make sure that computer's keyboard and the fingers position of the person working on it are comfortable and no stress is felt on the shoulders while the fingers are busy typing. The chair should be in alignment with the keyboard and keyboard should be adjusted just in front of computer screen, better in line with the center of computer. The screen of the computer should be in straight line and height with eyes of the operator. In seeing the screen, if the neck of operator is bending a little downwards or bending a little upwards, there may be problems in the neck after long use of computer. The best posture of neck is found out after ten minutes of use of computer. If you feel the strain in the neck muscles, you need a change in alignments. Any of these mentioned misalignments could lead to difficulties. (Please see 'Guidelines for those who work on computers' earlier in this for complete details)

Q.3. In spite of all the above precautions taken on the computer table, if someone complains that he or she suffers from neck pain not in the office but while going to home and taking rest. What can be done in such a case?

Answer: This is a case needing help of the doctor, who may take some X-ray to find out the exact cause of pain. If the pains are not of chronic nature and do not persist over the next day, it is a case which can be dealt properly by the physical therapy.

Q.4. If the choice is Homoeopathy for treating neck pain, what to tell the Homoeopath?

Answer: In case you have decided to visit a Homoeopath, there will be lot of questioning from him but the pertinent case of neck pain has to be told first in the following manner:

What is your profession? Are you an office worker, a computer-worker, a shopkeeper or a person doing work relating to manual exertion. By manual, it is not loading or unloading goods on the head but it is also the job requiring continuous neck movement like the job of driver, job of salesmen who drive scooters, bikes and cars etc. during their routine of work.

- Did the pain occur after an accident or a fall?

- How did the pain start?

- What is the movement that makes the pain worse and what is the posture that makes the pain relieved?

- The part of the neck that gives more of pain and does it radiates to other parts of the body, say shoulders or arms, hands etc?

- What is the type of pain, drawing, stitching, burning, stinging etc.?

- Any feeling of weakness of body associated?

- Sensation as if pricking of needles or feeling of numbness of the neck?

- If feeling of numbness, is it extending to other parts of the body?

- Is the neck stiff or there is mobility and whether upon mobility only, the pain occurs?

- Do you get this sort of pain frequently or was it the first time the pain occurred?

Q.5. Is exercise of neck essential especially when there is lack of time for a today's busy person? Will medication only help?

Answer: Continuous poor posture of neck cause undue strain on the muscles and ligaments. The result is that the ligaments become elongated and any further abnormal mechanical strain becomes the cause of many more symptoms. If there is no exercise on the part of the person getting bouts of neck pain and also that he is weak in body structure, he is vulnerable to mechanical strain than the one with a normal muscular build. The office worker or the person working on computer has his spinal muscles slack and weak due to his unstrenous job. If this man being of weak structure tries to lift something heavy or does heavy gardening work, he become more vulnerable to strains and pains than the person who is well build and does regular exercise. Daily exercise means that the muscles are in good shape.

Exercise, even if given very less time but regularly, has no equal to ward off not only neck pain but other ailments also. During the spells of neck pain, it is the doctor who decides whether you need exercise or not. The need for daily and normal exercises is another aspect of keeping whole body fit and it is up to the individual to fashion his life in the pattern he desires, the healthy one or otherwise. Time is never available for the man. It has to be snatched out of routine work. *A friend of mine, Mr. K.P.Dattaburman of Jaipur is a retired Drilling Engineer and son of a reputed doctor. He has a different logic on snatching time for exercises. It is worth mentioning here. He says, "A man has twenty four hours at his disposal and even if he can spare one minute in one hour for body exercise, the time of twenty four minutes is sufficient to keep a man live long and remain healthy."*

The medication does help relieve the pain but after the pains have subsided or gone, it is better to resume exercises, if advised by the doctor.

Q.6. Is there any restriction in diet-intake?

Answer: If the neck pains are due to rheumatic or gout factor, the doctors generally advise the patients to avoid meat and drinks. No doubt, food has a great role to play in eliminating pains and diseases. If our bowels were cleared, there would not be any distention and uprising of gases. Eructations and gases make a different type of pressure on the organs and the muscular network. Neck is no exception. It is the unity of body with all organs working separately but effects are united. If abdomen is upset the whole body is likely to suffer. Non-vegetarian food is not the order of the day and many people in western countries are leaving non-vegetarian food although they are born non-vegetarians. The story is different in India where people are born vegetarians and switchover to the other side only due to a misconceived theory of health-maintenance. People having neck and back pains should have more vegetarian diet including green vegetables, fruits and plenty of salad in the food. The water should also be taken in plenty so that the kidneys are flushed. The fruits, vegetables and grams compensate for vitamins and minerals besides helping the bowel flushing. (Please read instructions under heading 'Diet suggestion for patients of cervical spondylosis')

Q.7. Does tension have any impact on cervical spondylosis?

Answer: Research indicates that we attract almost all the diseases through our inappropriate method of handling the tensions, which act like magnets for diseases. Under the tension regime in the body, the act of tension releases many harmful toxic chemicals stored in our body causing fatigue, pain and disease. Tensions and worries tighten the muscles of the neck and upper back and shoulders and this aggravates the pain by increasing the lesion at the lever of cervical spine. It is very difficult to deal with tensions but once a man knows the way out, he gets free from pains as well. The best way out is to expose your problems to your friends, relatives or write down the problems to find out a solution. In responses to tensions, we are uneducated. Repressing the tension and worry will not save us from pain. On the other hand, swallowing in tension make us face external situations that confirm what we are experiencing. Avoiding the tensions, ignoring them, denying them or comparing them with the tensions of other persons are not the solutions. This is just like a mouse shutting eyes and avoid running after it sees the cat. Tensions do bring pains but they have a purpose to come. Tensions are meant to draw your attention to the unacceptable and your need to call for action. If you do so bravely and face the situation, tensions will not cause pains in your neck. (Please see heading 'Stress - a cause of cervical spondylosis')

Q.8. Do you advise avoiding sexual intercourse during the spells of neck pain?

Answer: Yes, during the spells of neck pain or lumbar region pain, sexual intercourse should not be carried out. There are some rules of this act. When the pain is not there, sex can be enjoyed but it should be during night so that a rest is obtained after this. There should be interval of at least three hours after dinner otherwise gout, rheumatism, lumbago etc. can aggravate, if existing. For the male patients of cervical spondylosis, the pose of sexual intercourse should not be man over the woman with his face downwards. It is better to go in for lateral position with man and woman on their sides or woman lying above the man with her face downwards. According to old sayings, it is not advisable to have intercourse in these positions but for the men suffering from neck pains, it could be a relief. For the female patients of cervical spondylosis, the former pose of man sleeping over the woman facing downwards is advisable. Do not enjoy sex with menstruating, pregnant or a diseased lady. Enjoy sex with wife.

Q. Do you advise avoiding sexual intercourse during the spell of ill-health?

CHAPTER 8

HOMOEOPATHY IN CERVICAL SPONDYLOSIS

THE FIRST question is why homoeopathy? It is not that homoeopathy is very popular and you have no other choice for any alternative system of medicine. It is not that the conventional system of medicine, allopathy, has totally turned you down. You did get the relief by allopathic medicines, by the physiotherapy methods suggested and the short time taken to get cure, may be it is temporary. All this benefited your body since your pains are over and whenever the pains occur again, you know the medicine, and the pain killer tablets and you take the same. The pain again subsides. Where is the need for shifting to homoeopathy then?

The one of the reasons to shift to homoeopathy is your inquisitive nature. The second reason is that you want to see if better results can be achieved without repeating the medicines. You desire a permanent relief. You have also option of Ayurveda but you feel that the cost of medicines is too high in comparison to homoeopathic medicines. So the third reason is the medicines are affordable and treatment costs less. The fourth reason is that there is no side effect as is found in conventional drug therapy.

HISTORY OF HOMOEOPATHY

Now you know the reasons to shift to Homoeopathy but what is homoeopathy? You must know its history first.

The oldest link and origin of homoeopathy relates to the era of fifth century BC (470-400) when a doctor called **Hippocrates, the father of medicine** invented two methods of healing, the 'contraries' and the 'similars'. There was a misconception those days that the ailments or illness was the punishment from the Gods. According to him, 'every disease has its own nature and arises from external causes, from cold, from the sun, from changing winds and that our nature is the physician of our diseases'. His very theory that diseases can be cured by 'similars' was not accepted then and it remained in dormant stage for thousands of years.

A German doctor, Paracelsus (1493-1541) went against the winds of his times. He saw the great earth as a chemical laboratory and identified the value of chemical experiments in medicines, both as the reason for understanding physiological processes and as a source of medicinal preparations. **Paracelsus was called the father of chemistry** because he desired to treat illness through pharmaceutical means. He made his study to base upon the animals and minerals and rallied against those who believed that contraries cured. *He turned to German folk medicine, which believed in 'like curing like' or that the poison that causes a disease should become its cure.* In this process, he found that giving smallest dose of poison could cure the disease. This was not the law of cure in actual meaning, which was exposed by another doctor after more than two hundred years.

It was Samuel Hahnemann of Germany (1755-1843), **the father of Homoeopathy** who made a history of change in treatment. He qualified as a doctor in 1791 and practiced medicine for about nine years. He became disillusioned by the cruel and ineffective treatments of his time (blood-letting, purging, poisonous drugs with horrendous side effects). He had an inordinate thirst for knowledge and his greatest talent was for learning languages, mathematics, geometry and botany. In his routine work of translating, he came across translation of a book, 'Treatise on Materia Medica' by Dr. William Cullen. Cullen wrote about Cinchona's (a herb) ability to cure malaria. Following his 'like cure like' principle, he took this herb and experienced all symptoms of malaria. This meant that cinchona produced in a healthy person the symptoms of malaria, the very disease that it was known to cure. This discovery paved a way for homoeopathic doctrine. Durings the next six years, Hahnemann conducted many provings on his family and friends and also studied accounts of the symptoms by the victims of accidental poisonings. In his further practice he looked for the *similimum* - the remedy whose 'symptom picture' most matched that of his patients. His colleagues ridiculed him but he continued his efforts. It was unheard in those days to give a single remedy when other conventional doctors made fortunes by mixing numerous substances, many of which were highly noxious. He used smaller and minimum doses for his patients. In 1810, he published his first edition of 'The Organon', which later ran into six editions. This book is supposed to be the 'Gita' of Homoeopathy.

Hahnemann was apparently a man with irritating nature with an antagonism but in spite of this, he had many followers who converted from allopathy to homoeopathy. **Dr. Constantine Herring** (1800-80) was his first follower. It was he, who was told to write a paper disproving Hahnemann's theory but while studying 'Organon', he gave credit to the theory of medicine proved by Hahnemann. He was successfully treated by Homoeopathy for inflammation of his hand that threatened amputation. He was thus totally convinced about Homoeopathy. It was he who made a proving of a snake poison, Lachesis.

After Herring, his next follower was **James Tyler Kent** (1849-1916) of America. His wife fell seriously ill and was treated by homoeopathy successfully. He was a man with a high moral sense and remarkable energy for writing. Kent's books are dogmatic, like Hahnemann's later works. He advocated use of very high potencies of medicines but like Hahnemann, his emphasis was on low potency like 30. He developed constitutional remedies and wrote many books of which his Materia Medica, Repertory and Philosophy are even used today by all. Those doctors who use high potencies of medicines and follow Kent's methods of prescribing are known as Kentians, a term that speaks of high caliber of a man, he was.

Homoeopathy is now popular not only in USA, Britain but in Asia as well, right from India to Pakistan, Bangladesh to Nepal and Sri Lanka. It is now recognized as official branch of medicine in India.

THE HELP OF HOMOEOPATHY

How can homoeopathy help in a case of cervical spondylosis? What is the duty of the homoeopath when the patient has come to him? The first duty is to assure the patient that the homoeopathic treatment will certainly make a dent in the followed procedure and betterment is surely expected. The main worry of the patient is that he has to take the medicines of the allopathic system whenever the pains occur and there is no permanent solution except surgery in some cases. It is the duty of the homoeopath to make the patient understand that a cure is possible in this discipline. For achieving the confidence of the patient, the doctor has to make a brief speech on the system of homoeopathy as to how it works. The patient has to be told in the following fashion.

THIS THEORY OF HOMOEOPATHY IS FOR A LAYMAN TO UNDERSTAND BEFORE TREATMENT

"Health is a state of balance and the disease is the result of weakness of the body's energy or vital force or the 'Aatmik Shakti'. Once the vital force gets diminished, the body reflects the same in any of the diseases and one of them is cervical spondylosis. The treatment is, therefore, aimed at strengthening the vital force so that the body itself heals the ailment. The symptoms of the disease are main features over which the medicines are selected. The remedies are based upon the theme that substances which produce same symptoms when these substances are given to a healthy person. When these substances in the form of remedy are given to the sick person,

having the same symptoms, which a healthy person produced, the healing takes place. The principle is 'like cures like' (law of similars). The remedies are made from herbs, plants, minerals, animals and other substances. The substances are repeatedly diluted, shaken or succussed by which the power of the substance is increased or call it that the substances are potentized. Potentization is nothing but increasing the invisible power of the substance. This sort of invisible power or energy stimulates the weak vital force because of the fact that it is of the same nature of which the patient suffers. It will nourish the vital force and restore the body to harmony. A homoeopath selects the remedy after checking with symptoms of the body and name of the disease is of no use to him. It is these symptoms, which enables him to choose the right remedy. If a patient of cervical spondylosis has ill temper, irritable behavior, talks very fast, has red, wild and staring eyes and cannot stand the sun-heat and his face a red color, his remedy is Belladonna. But this is not all; every person has a different remedy because different people have different symptoms. In spite that the patient has above symptoms but he lacks in thirst and is very restless or has his tongue with a white coating, the remedy will differ. Similarly, if a patient having urticarea has no thirst and a patient having the same disease has thirst with restlessness, the remedy will differ although the name of the disease is same i.e. urticarea. (Apis and Rhus tox.). In cervical spondylosis or in any disease, the whole base is symptoms and it is the skill of the homoeopath to understand and interpret the symptoms and select a remedy."

SOME CONFUSIONS REGARDING HOMOEOPATHY

Those who come to the rescue of homoeopathy have some confusion. Let us clear those confusions first to enable us proceed further.

CONFUSION-I, IS IT SAFE?

Yes, it is very much safe and free from side reactions but let me clear that it is not safe if the doctor is inexperienced. Please note that Kent, of whom we already read, said that he would rather share a room with a nest of vipers than be subjected to the administration of an inexperienced homoeopath.

If someone takes a wrong medicine over a period of time, there is possibility of proving the medicine. He will suffer from the symptoms the medicine is supposed to induct and the cure will not be there.

It is not safe if the patient does the medication by himself, after knowing the name of the medicine prescribed by the doctor.

Over-use of a remedy is also not safe.

CONFUSION-II, IS IT SUPPRESSION?

Homoeopathic medicines do not cause suppression. Suppression is uncommon in homoeopathy but is possible if the doctor does not give oral medicines and directly goes in for local applicants or allows allopathic creams (cortisone for ex-

ample) in skin diseases. Allowing application of allopathic oint-
ments and giving homoeopathic medicines internally may eliminate the skin disease temporarily but the disease will return.
Poor choice of remedy also leads to suppression.

CONFUSION-III, IS IT PLACEBO EFFECT?

Some people believe that homoeopathic remedies do have
placebo effect. A placebo is a pill without medicine. If you want
to check its potential, give it to a person having non-bleeding
head injury or in earache/toothache. The pill would not relieve
the pains. Only a right selected remedy would work in these
cases. Homoeopaths are utilizing placebo when high potency
dose is inducted to the patient and repetition is not desired. In
between the interval of high dose and time of next induction,
placebo is used so that the patient is satisfied that he or she is
taking medicine continuously.

CASE TAKING IN CERVICAL SPONDYLOSIS

There is nothing special while taking a case of cervical
spondylosis. In each case, there has to be complete agreement
with the procedure laid down by the great master in aphorism
84 of the Organon. This has been fully explained by J.T. Kent
in his book 'Lectures on Homoeopathic Philosophy'. Here is
my interpretation.

HOW TO RECORD THE CASE?

Case taking of the cervical spondylosis patient needs a lot of experience and training. This cannot be achieved by reading books only because the books will only provide basic knowledge and the method to take up the case. This means the process of knowledge will be in terms of rules. The actual learning comes from training from an experienced Homoeopath after one completes his or her BHMS. Initially one has to watch the proceedings of taking up acute and chronic cases, note down the impressions and then comes the questions and clarifications to be asked from the trainer Homoeopath. One has to interpret the uttering of the patient and conclude the symptoms as narrated by the patient. This, once written in one's own language needs a checking by the trainer. The main goal of the interview of the patient is to reach a totality of symptoms. To reach this goal needs lot of time and skill. Homoeopathic case taking is really an art.

Hahnemann has detailed the case taking in aphorism 100 in a very sensible manner as follows:

"...The novelty or peculiarity of a disease of that kind makes no difference either in the mode of examining or of treating it, as the physician must anyway regard the pure picture of every prevailing disease as if it were something new and unknown, and investigate it thoroughly for itself, if he desire to practice medicine in a real and radical manner, never substituting conjecture for actual observation, never taking for granted that the case of disease before him is already wholly or partially known, but always carefully examining it in all the phases." (Organon of Medicine:S. Hahnemann)

Now read this statement and you will be aware that the

doctor should never be prejudiced. J.T. Kent, in his book, 'Lectures on Homoeopathic Philosophy' elaborates on aphorism 100 of his master Hahnemann. What a great contribution Kent has made towards the rules of Homoeopathy in his own language interpreting the aphorisms in his novel method so that the followers get a clear picture of what Hahnemann intends to say. Here is Kent's summary of aphorisms 100.

"Keep that in your mind, underscore it half a dozen times with red ink, paint it on the wall, put an index finger to it. One of the most important things is to keep out of the mind, in an examination of the case, some other case that has appeared similar. If this is not done, the mind will be *prejudiced* in spite of your best endeavors. I have to fight that with every fresh case I come to. I have to labor to keep myself from thinking about thing I have cured like that before, because it would prejudice my mind.

SUGGESTED STEPS FOR EXAMINING THE PATIENT AND CASE RECORDING

■ As we said, case-recording is an art and one has to observe all *the preliminaries including interrogation, inspection, palpation, percussion, auscultation and special examination of the patient recording the name, age, gender, profession, and disease history.*

■ Let the patient narrate his or her complaints. Write down the complaints turn by turn and leave some space between each complaint so that you can write further on that particular complaint when you want an answer later.

- Write the complaints right from beginning to the day of patient's coming to you i.e. make a sequence.

- After you have written the history as above, now pay attention to the constitutional make-up of the patient. These are of three types, the structure of the patient, the mental make-up or emotional state and patient's place of living (damp house, hilly terrain, ill-ventilated house etc.)

- Enquire about the old history of patient's family like Tuberculosis, Asthma, Rheumatism, Cancer, Epilepsy, Diabetic, Cardiac problems etc.

- Now come to the physical examination. Check the pulse, temperature, respiration, inability to sit or stand for a longer time etc.

- Start checking from the head downwards. The patient's face will tell the mental condition as to whether he or she is worried, angry, depressed or frustrated. Note if there are black spots beneath the eyes or much below the facial line, yellow color of eyes, whitish skin of face, heaving long sighs by the patient with the result of inflation of nasal cavity, wrinkles on the forehead, ulcers, eruptions, pustules on the face.

- Inspect the shoulders, arms, neck, the dorsal region and the lumbar region. Now feel the carotid pulsation, dilatation of the veins, inflammation, bulging of skin and bones at the back and skin disease on any of the above organs.

- See the chest and back for any rickets (children) or emphysema (here the chest is protruded outside). Place your hand on the chest or back spreading it here and there to locate any bony change or pathological change. Ribs and clavicles must be checked for any inflammation or tumor etc.

- Now go in for percussion. Place your left hand middle finger on the chest or back of the patient and tap the finger with the help of your right hand index fingertip. The resonance will give a different sound of vibrations; dullness etc. It is a clue towards the condition of lungs. The tapping should be systematic. First tap the upper part of chest's right side and then the left side. Similarly tap the parts in the middle part of chest, right and left and finally the lower part of the chest, right and left.

- Now with the help of stethoscope, check the heart and lungs. The lungs need the same systematical examining i.e. upper, middle and lower parts of the chest or back, both right and left.

- X-ray and laboratory tests as needed are additional assets.

We should agree that a part of the above examination is for the allopathic nature of complaints. This examination gives us a little knowledge about the disease so far as homoeopathic treatment is concerned. Now we come to the questionnaire for the doctor. He should put the following questions:

- What are the foods that aggravate the condition? What about appetite, thirst, liking of salt or sugar etc., cravings and aversions?

- What about tiredness, sleeplessness, restlessness, dreams, peculiar trends during sleep, wants to keep the body covered or wants windows open etc.?

- What about sexual desires, aversions and any peculiar obsessions about sex-acts?

- What about emotions, phobia, fears, anxiety, concentration of mind, forgetfulness, delusions, mental symptoms and memory etc.?

■ What about menstrual functions, birth of babies, abortions, leucorrhoea and pains in the uterus region?

■ What about the various systems of body including stomach, abdomen or liver disorders, nature of urine, stool and associated complaints, burning of extremities, sweating, skin eruptions, dandruff, joint pains, respiratory problems, and endocrine or circulatory disorders?

■ What about the condition of health and its changes during day or night or particular seasons?

All the above questions should not be put directly to the patient but make your questions in such way that they appear indirect. Let the patient tell his or her sufferings of his/her own. For example, if the condition about menses is to be enquired, simply ask, what about the menses? Never say, "Are your menses profuse, scanty, irregular and so on"? Just say, "How about menses"? In all cases, such questions should be avoided which have a simple answer, yes or no.

THE SECOND PRESCRIPTION

Once the homoeopathic medicine has been given and some results have been noted, it is better to evaluate the same for the second prescription. For this note the changes in the appetite of the patient, digestion, stool habit, skin eruptions, cycle of menstruation, sexual urge and mental state. Such changes lead to correct second remedy change in the potency of the remedy. There are many types of patients. Some will come and report that after taking of your homoeopathic medicines, his or her palms and soles have started burning. Now have a check on the past history of the patient, whether he/she had this problem before taking of allopathic drugs. If it has returned, you are on the right path. Consider the same medicine on a higher potency level or think of a complementary to see the results, which will be positively be on the amelioration side. If there are some new complaints upon taking the homoeopathic remedy, note these and change the prescription according to the new symptoms. If the patient feels no change in his/her condition after taking homoeopathic medicine but the patient reports 'feeling good or general well-being feeling', the doctor should think that he is on the right path. There is no need for changing the prescription and Sac-lac can be recommended.

CHAPTER 9

CAUSATION FACTOR OR HOMOEOPATHIC ETIOLOGY IN NECK PAIN

S TUART CLOSE in his book, 'The Genius of Homoeopathy', has defined the causation factor in diseases.

He states, " The science of logic has an important relation to medicine in the matter of assigning the causes of disease, upon which, as far as possible, treatment is based. If treatment is to be governed to any extent by the idea of removing or counteracting the effects of the cause of the disease, it follows that success will depend upon correct conclusions as to what constitutes the cause or causes. Many, if not most, of the mistakes and failures in medical treatment are due to the failure to comprehend and correctly apply the principle of logic known as the

Law of Causation. Every one is quite ready to agree that every effect must have a cause. But investigation shows that very few seem to know, or, if they know, make use of their knowledge of the fact, that every effect has a number of causes, all of which must be taken into consideration if correct conclusions are to be formed."

He further gives reference of a scientist, Mill, on system of Logic, "The theory of induction is based upon the notion of cause. The truth that every fact, which has a beginning, has a cause and is coextensive with human experience. The recognition of this truth and its formation into a law, from which other laws are derived, is a generalization from the observed facts of nature, upon which all true science is based."

What Stuart Close has described on the law of causation is not a new phenomenon but development of Hahnemannian philosophy. As a matter of fact, other renowned homoeopaths of the era during and after Hahnemann not only followed his doctrine but also polished it, reviewed it and presented in such a manner so that it is clear to the next generation of homoeopaths. There are different interpretations from different scholars but the theme and contents remained the same.

Any disease including neck pain has to be effect of some cause. Without a cause, no one gets angry. Without fire around, there is no smoke. So, there has to be relation between the effect and cause. It cannot be said that the effect will be soon or immediate after the cause has occurred. This may be at a later stage. You must have noticed that old injuries healed with orthodox system of medicines sometimes emit pains after a very long time when even the injury has been forgotten. From individual to individual it varies. In Homoeopathy the causation has been considered to be very important clue for selection of a right remedy. Although every doctor belonging to any branch of medicine first enquires about the cause of ailments yet keen interest is taken in Homoeopathy to stress upon the cause of the ailment. It may be noted that the allopathic system of medicine claims the cause of disease to be effect of bacteria, viruses, parasites and other micro -organism. The biochemistry suggests the cause to be imbalance of body fluids, disturbance in metabolism and variations in cellular products. The Ayurveda believes that there is imbalance of Vata, Pitta or Kuff in the body as the cause of diseases.

It is not always true that the patient tells the cause. Actually he or she wants to know the cause of disease, if the disease is of chronic nature. Every patient is curious to know about the nature of disease and the cause of the disease. It is but natural. It depends upon the doctor from whom the patient enquires about the cause. If the patient is with the dentist, he will tell a headache to be on account of dental caries or toothache. If the patient is with ENT specialist, he will tell a headache to be due to ear, nose or throat problems. Similarly a heart specialist or a lungs specialist will narrate the causes of headache relating to their field of specialty. Homoeopaths are not trained as specialist of particular organs of body and they deal the person as a whole. For them the body is a unit without any compartmental treatment.

Homoeopathy does not abide by above reasons. It goes by the actual causes, be they are **exciting cause, maintaining cause or fundamental cause** as noted from the narration of the patient. What are these exciting, maintaining or fundamental causes? Let us have a look.

- If a patient of cervical spondylosis says that he got drenched in rain, the remedy is selected basing this drenching as a main cause. *This will be under exciting cause category.* Drenching is an external stimuli here.

- If the patient comes and reports that he gets the neck pain due to his professional reasons, say working on computers etc., this is *maintaining cause.*

- If the patient reports that his neck pain is from a long time and that it never ceases completely, there may be some organic reason or internal derangement. This is *fundamental cause.*

In all the above causes, the level of vital force is involved and the remedy has to base upon totality of symptoms including causes. There has to be a state of harmony of the vital force with the cause. If the doctors remove the external cause or the reaction of stimuli without looking into the internal derangements, the disease may return. This also means that the disease has taken its root deep inside the body. Take the example of allergic Asthma. If the cause is not only external stimuli or allergy, there may come some skin rashes or eczema, or there may be discharges etc. This can also be said suppression. What does this mean? It shows that the medicines given have suppressed the primary disease because it had no capacity to reach the internal derangements. If this type of suppression occurs, *it means the disease is of chronic nature.*

MATERIA MEDICA OF CAUSATION

Here is a study of some medicines, which can be considered

if the causation symptoms agree with the symptoms of the disease.

ABROTANUM

If the neck pain is of rheumatic nature and it has occurred after sudden checking of diarrhea by some medicines or checking of any type of secretions.

ACONITE

If the cause is exposure to dry cold wind, north or west winds, experiencing chill after perspiring or suppression of sweat and from any type of anger or shock.

ACTAEA RACEMOSA

If fright, anxiety or mental strain, exertion and child bearing are the reasons, this remedy is useful. If menses are delayed or suppressed and if the cause is rheumatism due to excessive use of typewriter or computer or sewing machine, this medicine is quite effective.

AGARICUS

This remedy can be used when there is nervous weakness after consumption of alcohol, if the pain has occurred before a thunderstorm and after eating or after coitus.

AESCULUS

When the aching started from walking or long standing or after eating, this can be used.

ANACARDIUM

After a hot water bath, if the neck pain has been experienced, this remedy is useful.

ARNICA

If the neck pain is due to bad effects of mechanical injury or too much of exertion, retention of urine after labor and due to taking liquors, this remedy has no equal.

ASARUM EUROPAEUM

When even the linen collar of the shirt causes irritation on the neck skin and sounds of others are felt penetrating, this remedy is useful.

AMMONIUM CARB

If the patient is leading sedentary life, gets the pain after smelling strong odors or after a bath, this remedy can be used.

BAPTISIA

When the patient gets the pain due to exposure to humid heat or fog, this remedy is of use.

BELLADONA

Diseases from drafts of cold air and hair cut are the reasons for giving this remedy.

BRYONIA

Complaints from disappointment, mortification and anger and when the neck pain has started in hot season after cold days, this remedy is useful. Also when the pain is the outcome of suppressed discharges and menses or after the diarrhea during hot season, this remedy is beneficial.

CALCAREA CARBONICA

Neck pain due to defective assimilation and imperfect ossification is one reason while the other reason is when the patient has been standing in cold damp places of work or doing work in cold water.

CAUSTICUM

When the pain is due to long lasting grief and sorrow, say a death of relative, or when there is loss of sleep, the patient is having night watching, experiencing sudden emotions of fear, anger or joy, after whooping cough and disturbed functional activity of brain or spinal cord or exhausting diseases and feeling of never been well since an attack of burns, this remedy is of immense use.

CHELIDONIUM

When the cause of pain is some malignant ulcer beneath neck or the patient suffers from liver or lung disease as well and the change of climate brings the pain, this remedy is of benefit.

COCCULUS

Cocculus is a wonderful remedy when the neck pain is due to riding in a carriage, rail, car or boat or patient is a drunkard or has loss of sleep due to night watching and the cause is bad effect of grief and anger.

COLOCYNTH

Anger with indignation, disappointment, pains after diarrhea and suppressed menses are the reasons for giving this medicine.

CONIUM

If the neck pain is the result of a blow or fall, after the suppression of menses when the patient has put hands in cold water and bad effects of sexual desires or excessive indulgence in sex.

DULCAMARA

Neck pain from sudden change in weather, catarrhal rheumatism due to exposure to cold, damp rainy weather, after malaria or rheumatic fever and bad effects of abuse of mercury are some of the reasons for giving this remedy.

GELSEMIUM

When the pain is due to nervous affection as the result of onanism in both sexes, bad effect of fear, fright, flashing or exciting news and sudden onset of emotions, the remedy is useful.

IGNATIA

This remedy is very useful when the pains are due to continued grief, mental and physical exhaustion, anger and disappointed love, when the patient is constipated and habitual smoker or chews tobacco.

KALI CARB

When the pain is due to exposure to sun heat and loss of vital fluids from the body and the patient is anemic, this remedy is of good use.

KALMIA

When the patient has to work that involves leaning forward

or looking down continuously and gets the neck pain, this remedy can be used.

LYCOPODIUM

If the patients get the pain in neck after drinking liquor, after a bout of anger, disappointment, anger, fright, mental exertion, over lifting heavy weights, over eating, indulges in excessive sex, suffers from some deep seated disease, constipation since puberty or when away from home or when the patient eats too much of bread, onions, smokes and chews tobacco and as a result gets the neck pain, this remedy is of great use.

MAGNESIA PHOS

When the pain is due to uncovering and cold air, cold bathing, cold water washing, over study and mental strain, Magnesia phos is the answer.

MEDORRHINUM

When the neck pain is due to rheumatic and spinal cord derangements and there are some cysts or other growths in the body, this remedy can be used as intercurrent.

NUX VOMICA

When the cervical pain is for want of exercise and the patient has sedentary habits. Result of grief and anger, mental exertion, loss of sleep, sexual excesses, over eating, gastric upset, flatulence, highly spiced food, getting chilled and abuse of alcohol, tobacco, coffee and patent medicines are specific reasons for giving this remedy.

PHYTOLACCA

Rheumatic pains and neuralgia after syphilis, gonorrhea or abuse of mercury are the reasons for prescribing this remedy.

PARIS QUADRIFOLIA

When the pain in the neck is due to catarrhal complaints with stuffed feeling in the nose, and head symptoms are more marked, this remedy is useful.

RHUS TOX

When the neck pain is due to getting wet, especially after getting overheated, exposure to cold and dampness or lying on the damp floor, over exertion, trauma, taking bath in the cold water in summer, over lifting and sprains, this remedy is beneficial.

RHODODENDRON

If the neck pain is from thunderstorm, getting wet, cold and windy weather and the patient is of nervous nature, this remedy is useful.

SPONGIA

When the neck pain is from dry cold weather and the patient has cough from mental exertion as accompaniment of the pain, this medicine is of use.

SULPHUR

If the neck pain is due to suppressed eruptions of skin, hemorrhoids, discharges and vital fluids or when there is abuse of drugs, eating (over eating), becoming chilled, after debilitating diseases, from washing and bathing, drinking excessive liquor and abuse of metals, this wonderful remedy acts to the benefit of patients.

THUJA

When the neck pain is due to suppressed gonorrhea, abuse from tea, coffee, fats, tobacco, onions, sweets, drug containing sulpher and mercury, after taking vaccination, and excessive walking and riding, Thuja is useful.

REPERTORY OF CAUSATION OF NECK PAINS

Exertion from	Ant-c.
Chill from	Aco.ars., bry., colch., ferr-p., kalm.
Coffee from	Coff., nux-v.
Coition from	Con., kali-c., mag-m., nit-ac., sabal.

Cold from	Agar., am-c., cham., cist., kali-c., nat-m., nux-m., rhus-t., sabad.
Gonorrhoea after	Clem., con., cop., crot-h., daph., kalm., lyc., med., phyt., puls., sep., sulph., thuj.
Haemorroids	Abrot.
Malaria from	Aran., ars., chin., chinin-s., nat-m., stann.
Cloudy weather from	Calc-p., dulc., rhod., rhus-t.
Cold and damp weather from (stiffness)	Lach.
Cold and damp weather (general) from	Dulc., phyt., ran-b., rhod., rhus-t., verat.
Stormy weather from	Rhod., rhus-t.
Warm weather from	Colch., kali-bi.
Wine from	Led., mez., zinc.

Note

Leave aside the exciting cause or external stimuli, the other two causes mostly belong to chronic nature and for this we have to study the doctrine of chronic diseases as formulated by the great master. Hahnemann did identify that miasms are the fundamental causes of any disease. Once fundamental cause is removed, the body comes in harmony with vital force. What are miasms and their connection with neck pains, this we shall now study?

CHAPTER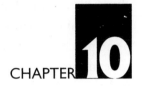

CERVICAL SPONDYLOSIS - A MIASMATIC STUDY

THE GREATEST asset to the era of Homoeopathy lies with the conception of miasmatic theory initiated by great master Hahnemann. Miasmatic theory has no connection with the chemical and mechanical activities or force of the body. This is the theory of an invisible vital force without which there would not be any organic chemistry. Hahnemann understood the wrong conception of the times in respect of medicines and revolted against it. He negated all the prevailing systems declaring them unscientific. According to him, the spring could not reach a higher level than the source. This is really true. Hahnemann reached the spring source and proved that the allopathic medicine system cannot reach the height of the spring i.e. homoeopathy. Now when we see back and watch the progress made by both the systems, we find that the allopathic system has not changed materially and that their modes and methods of procedure have changed. The allopathy has abandoned certain old values and methods and accepted new ways, which are also with certain drawbacks of side effects etc. On the other hand, Homoeopathy sails in the same boat having the same principles but with a refined out-look. Now Allopaths do agree to send their patients to the Homoeopaths, (Even if not openly, by hearsay) for treatment of warts, skin diseases and removal of kidney stones without operation. What I am pointing out is that a system without a law cannot be compared with a system having a fixed law.

Why a miasmatic study is required for treatment in Homoeopathy is a standing question among the learners? I quote here J.H. Allen from his book, 'Chronic miasms and Pseudo Psora' (B. Jain publishers - 1994) for a better understanding the theory of miasms.

"Someone may ask, why it is necessary for a true homoeopath to know about these chronic miasms. As long as he prescribes according to the law of similar, he cures the cases. There are many reasons why he should be able to distinguish their presence in the organism, whether it is psora, latent syphilis, especially the tubercular form, or whether it is sycosis. Dr. Herring, however, in his introductory remarks in the Organon (3rd American edition), thinks it not of vital importance: " What important influence can it exert whether a homoeopath adopt the theoretical opinions of Hahnemann or not, so long as he holds the principal tools of the master and the materia medica of our schools? What influence can it have, whether a physician adopt or reject the psoric theory, so long he always selects the most similar medicine possible." The last line is well timed: "*So long as he selects the most similar medicine possible*".

The fact is that we cannot select the most similar remedy unless we understand the phenomena of the acting and the basic miasms, whether we are conscious or unconscious of the fact. The curative remedy is but the pathopoesis of a certain pathogenesis of an existing miasm. The proving of the remedy would be very indefinite to us if the name were withheld from us. Suppose that you were making a proving of sulphur or aconite. Why, the first thing you would do, would be to ask for their names, you would say, I shall not attempt to use these remedies without knowing their names. So it should be with the disease-producing agent. We should know, not only the name of that underlying principle that fathers that phenomena with which we are so diligently and earnestly contending and combating. It is the difference between an intelligent warfare and fighting in the dark, it is no longer a battle in the mist. Again, suppose that we prescribe the similar remedy and have no knowledge of the law of action and reaction (or primary and secondary action), how can we watch the progress of a case without a definite knowledge of these disease forces (miasms), with their mysterious but persistent progressions, pauses, rests, forward movements, retreats, and attacks among unfamiliar lines, and of whose multiplied modes of action we have taken no cognizance? In fact we know nothing about the traits and characteristics of our enemy, is it possible to wage an equal warfare? Suppose that one would say that disease was due to bacteria, to a certain germ, to atmospheric conditions, to taking cold - facts to which the majority of diseases are attributed, would those facts assist us in the selection of the similar remedy? Would they help us to understand the phenomena of germ development, of taking cold? Why should he get a cold? Why should one have germs or be subject to atmospheric changes? Why should disease return in the same form or some diverse form? These are the things that disturb the mind of Hahnemann, and all this landed him to discover the psoric theory of the disease."

According to Allen, the doctors who select the similar remedies to cure their patients are not true healers of the sick because they are ignorant of the causes and effects of the disease.

IMPORTANCE OF MIASMATIC THEORY AND DISEASE

In Para 15 of the Organon, Hahnemann describes his theory of miasms, "The suffering of the immaterial vital principle which animates the interior of our bodies, when it is morbidly disturbed, produces symptoms in the organism that are manifest," and it is these morbidly produced symptoms that constitute what is known as disease in all multiplied forms, whether functional or structural. Knowledge of all miasmatic theory is complete knowledge of all that is known as disease, and beyond these symptoms there is nothing discoverable or recognizable as disease. This Hahnemann elaborates in Para 19 of Organon; "Disease is nothing more than changes in the general state of the human economy, which declare themselves as symptoms."

This also means that disease is the after effect (influence) of some subversive force, acting in conjunction with the vital force, subverting the action and changing the physiological momentum. Here Allen is again referred for his philosophical definition of disease, "*Disease is the totality of the effects, by which we recognize or perceive the action of a peculiar order of subversive forces upon an organism which has been exceptionally or specially adapted to, or prepared for their reception.*"

This statement makes the theory of miasms more near. A close study of the above statement draws a conclusion that disease is the vicarious embodiment of some miasmatic influence that has bonded itself with the life force, producing disease according to the type, as is seen in psora or any other of the chronic miasms.

It has been seen that a well-selected remedy given for the symptoms totally cures the case for time being. The symptoms are removed but after sometime, they return with same or more former force. This means that the disease has some deep roots in the body of the sufferer. The disease had been removed temporarily with the use of higher potency medicine but this time the return is with some change in expression of the symptoms. Most of the time these changes point to the order of the disease in the earlier stage. A man having a skin disorder gets cured but his early suffering asthma returns. When asthma is cured, his severe backache returns. What does all this show? What is the source of existence of diseases? It must be some latent, inherent, internal, pre-existing cause, having its habitat in the organism. Such habitat is not connected with the material body but with the dynamism or the life force. Thus it becomes a part of life force.

We talked of skin disease. Skin does not produce an eruption by itself, (leave aside the mechanical or chemical or traumatic reasons) and does not get a morbid state unless it is obliged by some previous perverted change of abnormal activity in the organism itself. An eruption is an expression that the disease inside has come out. The disease from a latent stage is now living and it certainly has a background of miasms through which it's opening had been possible. The background is psora, here.

THE THREE MIASMS

After twelve years of deep study on the patients, Hahnemann concluded that there are three basic miasms, which are the underlying causes of all chronic diseases. Further he pointed out that a patient may be a victim of one miasm or may have combination of miasms. As we discussed earlier, the first one is psora miasm. 'Psora' derived from Greek language means itch. As per Hahnemann, this is the earliest miasm affecting the mankind or human race with a most fundamental hidden element of debility or disease. It is this underlying debility, which gives rise to various other diseases. Hahnemann made a related history or link of diseases like diabetes, arthritis, cancer, mental diseases, epilepsy, etc. with *psora*.

The second miasm in the row is 'syphilitic' miasm with which the human race is affected. The name of the disease, 'syphilis' is considered to be one of the manifestations of this miasm. Besides this disease, there is a wide range of other disorders attached with this miasm. Hahnemann had formed an idea that those who suffered from syphilis miasm acquired this disease through exposure to the basic disease syphilis or it might have been by inheritance from an infected ancestor. This miasm runs from family to family of generations.

The third maism discovered by Hahnemann was the *sycosis* miasm. In Greek language, syco means fig. It is the manifestation of the disease gonorrhea, wither contacted by the patient or by one of the patient's ancestors.

On combinations of the miasms, Hahnemann is very clear and cites an example. If a person is weakened by the psora miasm but is also exposed to venereal diseases by one of his or her sins or sexual conduct, he or she is bound to be sick with the second miasm, syphilis. This combination of miasms then runs from generation to generation.

Can we say with authority that such and such disease by name is the outcome of psora, syphilis or sycotic miasm? No, we cannot say so because of severe intermingling of miasms at different stages of diseases. Let us see. We consider psora miasm responsible for itch or eczema, syphilis miasm exhibit ulcers and sycotic miasm, a disease of figs (skin disease) but this is proved that all three miasms can result in any pathological change. Cancer, diabetes, insanity or imbecility can arise from the last stage of any of the miasms or from any combination of them.

MIASMATIC REMEDIES FOR CERVICAL SPONDYLOSIS

The cervical spondylosis can be categorized under the main disease rheumatism. *For rheumatism, the hidden miasms behind are psora and sycosis.*

SOME ANTIPSORIC MEDICINES

Alumina, Aloes, Ambra grisea, Anacardium, Antim crudum, Apis, Argentum nitricum, Arsenic alb., Arsenic iod., Aurum metallicum., Baryta carb., Belladona, Acid benzoic, Berberis vulgaris, Borax, Bufo, Calcarea group of medicines, all Carbons, Capsicum, Ferrum group of medicines, Heper sulpher, Iodium,

Kali group of medicines, Lachesis, Ledum, Lac caninum, Lycopodium, Magnesia group of medicines, Natrum group of medicines, Acid nitric, Petroleum, Phosphorus and its acid, Platinum, Plumbum, Psorinum, Pyrogen, Silicea, Sepia, Sarsa, Secale, Selenium, Stannum, Staphysagria, Sulphur, Acid sulphuric, Tarentula, Theridion, Tuberculinum and Zincum metallicum.

SOME ANTI-SYCOTIC MEDICINES

Argentum metallicum, Argentum nitricum, Acid benzoic, Agaricus., Anacardium, Antim crudum, Antim tart, Arsenic alb, Apis, Asterias rubens, Aurum metallicum, Baryta carb, Bryonia, Berberis vulgaris, Calcarea ars., Calcarea sul., Carboanimalis, Carbo veg, Causticum, Clemitis, Colchicum, Dulcamara, Acid fluor., Iodium, Kali bich., Kali carb., Kali iod., Kali sul, Lycopodium, Lachesis, Magnesia carb., Magnesia mur., Magnesia phos., Medorrinum., Mezerium, Acid muriaticum, Natrum ars., Natrum carb., Natrum mur., Natrum sulph., Nitric acid, Phosphoric acid, Phosphorus, Psorinum, Pyrogen, Phytollacca, Pulsatilla, Sarsaparilla, Sepia, Silicia, Staphysagria, Thuja and Tuberculainum.

IMPORTANT NOTE ON SELECTION OF REMEDIES FROM ABOVE CATALOGUE

The above catalogue serves the purpose **when the disease has gone deep into the system** and has many more symptoms along with cervical spondylosis. The selection of remedy should be made according to symptoms and depending upon the miasm to which the remedy belongs.

You will find that very important remedies like Bryonia, Rhus tox, Ruta, Colocynthis etc. have not been mentioned in the above group of remedies prominantly. Basically these medicines are **meant for acute conditions and give very good results.** Bryonia is mostly meant for complaints from change of weather from cold to warm, getting chilled, dryness and more of thirst. Pains are sore, stitching and bruised. If such acute conditions occur, Bryonia helps. Rhus tox is for complaints from getting wet, change of weather to cold, damp, getting chilled. On change of weather to the damp, Rhus tox patient will start to moan and complain. This is one of the most important remedies for rheumatic/arthritic remedies. Like Rhus tox, Ruta is a remedy for sprain. While the former is for damaged ligaments and later is for injuries to the tendons and the periosteum (covering on the bones). Colocynthis is one of the main colic remedies like Staphysagria and Dioscorea.

We should keep in mind between the acute and chronic condition of the disease before looking for miasmatic remedies.

Acute diseases are those, which have a sudden onset, keep a short duration and also have sudden outcome either a complete cure without treatment or death. So, we should say that acute disease is the one, which tends to cease. The acute diseases flare up by the latent chronic miasms due to some exciting causes. *Identification of miasms can help find out a right remedy in the group of medicines mentioned above.*

HOW TO IDENTIFY MIASMS IN CERVICAL SPONDYLOSIS?

PSORA

The basic feature of psora is hypersensitivity and reactivity. The patient is very sensitive and thinks too much. He or she has sweating in the morning, chilliness in the evening and feels hot in the night. The patient has voluptuous itching, burning in the skin and may have vesicular eruptions. His *latent symptoms* are many but pertaining to cervical spondylosis, these are easy fatigue, mentally and physically, restlessness at night while sleeping, frequent flashes of heat and cramps, vertigo aggravated by walking, chronic headache, all sorts of skin diseases, and *glandular swelling of neck.* Sulphur is the medicine to be given in between the main medicine depending upon the basis of totality.

SYCOSIS

The basic feature of sycosis is figwart like growth. The patient here is oversensitive to an extent that this leads to debility. In psora, the oversensitive leads to hyperactivity but in sycosis, it leads to debility, which in turn produces disorientation and complete imbalance in sensations and functions. His *latent symptoms* are slow in recovery in spite of medicines, warts and warty growths and moles, nails thick and ridged, fixed ideas and hair falling in circular spots. Spondylosis features contain rheumatic and gouty complaints, headache during night with neck pain, and the patient is anemic.

SYPHILIS

Syphilis is not related with spondylosis but in case of *mixed miasms, its identification should also be made. Totally exhausted person with exhausted system and over stimulated state of body is the main feature. Mentally dull, stupid, suspicious and morose. Deformities in neck region with atrophy and syphilitic eruptions, bone pains at night and destructions from the very beginning in any disease are latent symptoms.

---

*Knowledge of mixed miasms is not so clear. Their symptoms are in a confusing manner. There may be lot of symptoms and not a single one characterizing the patient. The modalities and generalities are masked. It is said that nosodes are beneficial in solving the puzzle of blended miasms.

2

PART

PART

2

CHAPTER 11

THERAPEUTIC SUGGESTIONS MATERIA MEDICA OF CERVICAL SPONDYLOSIS

ABROTANUM

THIS MEDICINE is to be thought over when the diarrhea or some other secretions have been suppressed by some medication from other system of medicines. Pain in shoulders, neck, arms with pricking and coldness of fingers. Pain aggravation with cold winds. Excessive pain before the swelling of neck commences. Neck pain alternates with hemorrhoids and with dysentery. Neck is felt very weak and one cannot hold head up. This remedy has a significant action on the nervous system and it can produce hyperemia and anesthesia besides that it has capability to act tremendously on the fibrous tissue, which in turn are responsible for initiating rheumatic diseases. There is defective assimilation, which produces weakness in the body.

ACONITE

Aconite is more suitable for acute than for chronic diseases. Suddenness of symptoms of neck pain with anguish and fear. Feels that he or she may die because of this pain. The complaints are brought from exposure to dry, cold winds or from checking of perspiration. Neck pain is worse during evening and night. There may be fever also with neck pain. If the disease has caused pathological changes, Aconite is not to be used. As a matter of fact, Aconite if not found useful after three days of use, should be discontinued. The remedy causes only functional disturbance and there is very little evidence of power to produce tissue change. The action is brief and shows no marked periodicity. The onset of neck pain is sudden and there may be some chill or alternative chilliness and fever with neck pain. Restlessness is noticeable in all the cases requiring the remedy. The patient cannot remain still and is constantly moving an arm, leg, neck or tossing in the bed, turning in the bed or grabbing the covers. The patient will give a hurry call to the doctor for his sudden neck pain, and anxiety will always be written on his face. Aconite is frequently overlooked in neuralgia of the extremities, especially the upper, with numbness of the limbs if the blood did not circulate freely and particularly if the neuralgia is the result of cold or a sudden check of perspiration. Acute muscular rheumatism sometimes calls for Aconite but it is seldom indicated in inflammation of the joints or neck.

Modalities: The neck pain is worse in the evening and night, from sun's heat, hot days and cold nights, dry cold winds and air, when under a warm cover, in a warm room, from lying on the affected side, tobacco, smoke, contact and even music. The pain is better open air, lying or sitting still, after the spell of perspiration and uncovering.

AESCULUS HIPPOCASTANUM

One of the best remedies for rheumatic pains. Most of its action is on the lower back and pelvic area but neck is not altogether eliminated in its affection especially when there is lameness in the neck and aching between the shoulders. Weakness in the spinal region is one of the indications. If the patient is suffering from venous statis, piles, varicose veins and feels better in summer than winter. The pain dart from left to right in the neck and walking aggravates the pains. When neck pain is associated with pain in the small of back or in the sacrum and hips.

Modalities: Walking aggravate the pain as stated above. It is more in the morning, after stools, after eating, stooping and when rising from the bed and after standing. Pain is felt better in the cool open air and summer season.

AGARICUS MUSCARIS

It is quite useful in rheumatic and neuralgic pains of neck. There is a feeling as if icy cold needles pierce neck. Twitching of cervical muscles is characteristic of Agaricus. The neck pain has sensitiveness of spine to touch especially in the dorsal region and if some pressure is applied with hands, it may produce involuntary laughter. The neck is stiff and sprained sensation in the whole of back with weakness of muscles. Spondylitis with pain in the left arm. When some exercise is done for neck, there is great weariness. Paroxysms of yawning accompany the neck pain. There is sleepiness after eating and once the patient sleeps, the twitching in the neck or eyes start. With pain in the neck, there is tingling and formication in the back with itching and biting. The general action of the medicine is on the nervous centers and upon the brain as there is action of alcohol. It shows more vertigo and delirium. Tremors and twitching of the eyelids characterize it. Over study and excessive brainwork produces neck pain. It is a valuable remedy for the people living in hill regions and who have bad effects of frostbite and chilblains.

Modalities: Worse from open cold air, cold weather, before a thunderstorm, after eating, after sexual intercourse and from pressure on spine. The neck pain is better while moving about slowly.

ANACARDIUM ORIENTALE

The rheumatic symptoms of this remedy are related to stiffness of neck and torticollis or wry-neck. There is tearing and sticking pain in between the shoulders and a feeling as if there is heavy load on the shoulders. Pain in the spine as if from a plug in it which goes deeper with any motion of the body. During the act of writing, the right arm aches and the fingers twitch with cramps. In general, the patient has impaired memory, brain-fag and absent-mindedness. The patient averts to work and has empty feeling in the stomach.

Modalities: Pain of neck is worse when hot fomentation is applied, on stepping hard and mental exertion. Pain is better from eating, sitting, lying on sides and rubbing.

ARNICA MONTANA

Arnica is best suited to red-faced plethoric persons who are extremely sensitive to mechanical injuries. It is a polycrest used very successfully in rheumatic affections of muscular and tendinous tissues of back, shoulders and hips. The pains are sharp, shooting, sprained and change places quickly. In the neck region, there is twitching pain on the left shoulder, which extends to middle finger. Pain begins low down from back to neck. Pain in the last cervical vertebra on bending head and there is tension felt in bending. There is pain also in the middle of spine when sitting as if the body is unable to carry weight of body. Pain between the scapulae is characteristic. The remedy is best suited to those who work or toil hard, lift heavy weights and get exposed to damp cold. It is most valuable in chronic cases of neck pain. When lying down, the bed feels too hard and changing positions of lying relieves neck pain. The head and neck of the patient are hot while the remaining body is cool.

Modalities: Pain in the neck is worse with least motion and touch, rest, drinking wine, in damp cold weather, in the evening, from blowing nose and even from speaking. Pain is better lying down, lying with head low, warmth, rubbing the neck and wrapping the neck warmly. If the patient walks in cold weather, the pains are less.

ARSENIC ALB.

It is *not a very effective remedy for rheumatic affections* but if the totally of symptoms indicate, it proves useful. Burning and tearing pain in the neck and neck is stiff as if bruised or sprained. There is drawing pain between the scapulae, which compels the patient to lie down. Pain in the neck and the side, the patient lies on. Best suited to broken down constitutions and patients who are weak, cold, pale, lean and appear bloodless. There is great anxiety, anguish and extreme restlessness. The neck and the body feel extremely cold.

Modalities: Worse from touch, at night, left side of neck, during rest. Better open air, motion, and pressure.

ASARUM EUROPOEUM

Tension, pressure and contractive sensation in the neck are chief symptom. There is a feeling that the whole body or single part of the body is being pressed together.

Modalities: Worse cold dry weather or dry weather. Better damp wet weather and wetting affected part i.e. neck.

AMMONIUM CARB

Dragging pains in the nape of neck and as if some ulceration is in the muscles. Sometimes shooting pains are felt in the neck and surrounding regions. Right side of the neck is more affected than left side.

Modalities: Pains worse in the evening, cold wet weather, washing, during 3-4 a.m. Pains better on lying on painful side, dry weather and heat of the bed.

BAPTISIA

When the underlying cause of neck pain is infection and disorganization of blood. The rheumatic symptoms are unbearable pain in the neck on moving the head. Muscles of neck are stiff and tired along with pain in the sacrum. Pain in the neck is worse stooping.

BELLADONNA

It is one of the best remedies in both acute and chronic rheumatism of inflammatory nature. The pains come suddenly and after a while cease suddenly. Wry neck (torticollis) and stiffness of neck with inflammation and swelling of glands are main symptoms. There is pain in the nape as if it would break and shooting pains in the region of second and third vertebrae (cervical) on erecting the neck. There is pressure on the dorsal region also and gnawing in the spine as if back would burst.

Modalities: Pain is worse at 3 p.m., night, by after midnight, lying down, touch, light, noise, drafts of air, cold, uncovering head, sudden change of weather from hot to cold, in hot seasons, hot sun, and pain is more on the right side of neck. Pains are better while sitting erect or standing, by warm applications, wrapping up, in a hot room and keeping head high.

BRYONIA ALBA

It is one of the best remedies for rheumatism both acute and chronic neck pains. There is pain and stiffness in the nape of neck and also stitches and stiffness in the small of back. The pains develop slowly and mostly on the right side of neck. It is best suited to persons of a dry, bilious and nervous constitution with irritable temperament, given to overeating and with a tendency to gouty and rheumatic diathesis.

Modalities: Worse pains in warm weather after a spell of cold weather, hot weather, warmth, suppressed perspiration, anger, wet weather, any type of motion, morning, 9 p.m., after eating, exertion and touch. Pains better by rest, lying on painful side, moderate pressure, and cold things.

CALCAREA CARBONICA

It is also considered one of the most useful remedies for arthritic and rheumatic affections of neck. Nape of neck stiff and rigid and pains are there as if the neck is dislocated. The neck pain starts when the cause is by lifting a weight. Cervical vertebrae feel loose and are painful on pressing the nape of neck.

Modalities: Pains worse from mental or physical exertion, ascending, cold in every form, water, washing, moist air, wet weather, change of weather, near or during full moon, standing, evening, after midnight, from working in water i.e. washing, straining from lifting, on awakening and early in the morning. Pains are better by lying on painful side, on rising, after breakfast, dry weather and sneezing.

CAUSTICUM

Pain in the nape of neck as from a bruise and painful stiffness between scapulae are two main symptoms for using this remedy. One cannot raise his hands above the head. The stiffness of neck is so acute that one can hardly move his head. there is acute and violent pulling in the joints of neck. The stiffness of neck is more when rising from sitting position. It is a deep acting remedy of a wide range and therefore has many symptoms, which should be noted when selecting this remedy for neck pain. It is more useful in chronic neck pains especially on right side.

Modalities: Pains worse in dry cold winds, in clear fine weather, cold air, motion of carriage, walking, after stools and at new moon time. Pains are better in open air, warmth, heat of bed, drinking cold water, stooping low and emission of flatus.

CHELIDONIUM

It is a great liver remedy but its rheumatic and arthritic diseases are invariably associated with hepatic derangements. There is drawing cramp like pain in the neck with head drawn to the left. Pain is also in the right neck muscles and the region of right clavicle. There is sharp stitching constant pain beneath right scapula as found in Bryonia.

CIMICIFUGA OR ACTAEA RACEMOSA

It is a valuable remedy particularly for women suffering from neck pains. It has a special affinity for the vertebral joints, large muscles of trunk, the cervical and three upper dorsal vertebrae. The remedy has a marked action on spinal nerves especially at the upper part as also on the cerebrospinal and muscular systems in nervous subjects particularly women who suffer from uterine and ovarian affections. Pain in the neck comes suddenly and like electric shocks. They are sharp and lancinating with a feeling of stiffness and retraction. The pain also wanders here and there around the neck but prefers left side of neck in most cases.

Modalities: Pains are worse at night, morning, motion, and cold and during menses. They are better at rest, warmth, and open air and after eating.

COCCULUS INDICUS

Cocculus is a better-known medicine or cerebrospinal system producing great weakness of the spine and paretic or spasmodic affections. On the neck, it has pain and stiffness in the muscles on movement of the neck and head. On yawning, the pain in the neck increases and when the patient leans backward, the pain is less. Movement of shoulders or when the hands are on work, the neck-pain and stiffness is more. There is pressure in the scapulae and nape of neck. It is best suited to children and women. The medicine is mostly employed in patients having journey sickness/vomiting when traveling in car, bus or train.

COLOCYNTH

It is a remedy, which has been considered very useful in treatment of rheumatic diseases especially right thumb, hip and muscles where severe and sudden pains occur. The neck pains are of tearing, drawing and burning nature. Left neck -muscles is affected where drawing pains occur. The pains are worse moving the head to left side and there is stiffness also felt when moving the head. Similar drawing pains are felt in the area of right scapula as if its nerves and vessels are under strain. The relief of pain is when the patient bends double. Pain comes in waves and is better from heat and pressure.

CONIUM

Conium is one of the best remedies for the spine. It is long acting and best suited to old persons, old bachelors, old maids and widows. The pain in the neck is cramp like and mostly come in night disturbing sleep especially when one is totally fatigued due to day's work. The pains may also be due to some blow or strain. There is vertigo felt when the patient turns his or her head sideways during sleeping position. A constant tension is felt in the neck always even after the pains cease.

Modalities: Worse when turning head sideways, at night, during rest, lying down, while eating, before and during menses, on starting to move the head and from continued motion. Pains are better when releasing the neck loose, motion, applying pressure, fasting and bending the body forward.

DULCAMARA

Not a prominent remedy for chronic neck pain but is useful when the pains are induced by or aggravated by damp cold or drenching. Torticollis (wry neck) with stiffness and lameness around the neck and shoulders are important symptoms.

GELSEMIUM

It is a beneficial remedy for neuralgic rheumatism. Deep seated dull aching in the muscles of neck. The neck feels bruised and there is sensation as if there is no muscular power in the neck. If the patient desires to move the neck, the muscles do not obey it instantly or we can say that there is in-coordination. Five 'D's are to be remembered for selecting this remedy. **D**ullness, **d**rowsiness, **d**izziness, **d**oddering (trembling), and **d**rooping of eyelids is the five symptoms leading to this remedy.

IGNATIA

This remedy has been used widely for neck pains especially when there is lack of sleep due to some grief. The pain is in small spots and stiffness is always there in the neck. The stitching pains are of the nature as if there had been dislocation or sprain in the joints of neck. The pains are worse in the morning, open air and after meals. Even smoking relieves the patient. The pains are mostly better during summer, warmth and walking.

KALI CARBONICUM

Like Ignatia, the patient suffers from depression but the sleep is easy in this remedy. The very characteristic stitching pains are felt in the neck with stiffness. A great deal of weakness follows. Sometimes numbness is also there and sometimes the neck feels paralytic. The pains are worse after coition, in cold season, after eating, at rest, on uncovering, in the morning about three AM, lying on the left side and bending backward. The neck pain is better in summer, warmth, during the day, when moving about or sitting and bending forward.

KALI NITRICUM

This remedy is meant basically for asthma and dropsical swelling of the whole body. If the patient suffers from asthma and has frequent neck pains, this remedy can be used. There are stitches between shoulder blades with tearing and sticking in shoulders and joints. The patient feels as if his hairs are being pulled while the pain in the neck remains.

KALMIA

Kalmia is considered a true rheumatic remedy foe neck pains if the pains are shifting from one side to the other. Actually it acts chiefly on the muscular and nervous systems with principal action on the heart. There is vertigo also with neck pains. One cannot touch the neck as the touching is extremely sore. The pains are neuralgic mostly on right side of neck with numbness and shift downwards. This shifting is rapid and sudden.

Modalities: The pains are worse by motion, exertion, and open air, looking down and bending forward. The pains are relieved when eating food and after urination.

LYCOPODIUM

Not a usual remedy for neck pain but if the other symptoms of the body agree, this works. There is pain in the neck with stiffness of left side, torticollis (wry-neck), burning pain between the scapulae as if hot coal has been placed at the neck. Pains come and go suddenly.

LACHNANTHES

It is a specific remedy for torticollis and rheumatic symptoms about the neck. Neck is drawn over to one side, mostly towards right in sore throat. There is stiffness of the neck and pain in the nape as if it is dislocated. While comparing this medicine, one should not forget the remedy Fel tauri for a comparison. The pain and stiffness of neck is more when the neck is either turned or moved backwards. The pain also extends towards head and travels to nose.

MAGNESIA PHOS

This remedy has a multiple use in treatment of spasmodic

pains associated with neuralgias and cramping. In whole of materi medica, there is no other remedy, which has a huge variety of pains. It is useful in all types of pains like shooting, stabbing, knife-like, stitching, piercing, cutting, sharp and like lightening, coming and going. In this remedy, the pains are better by application of warmth. One cannot rely upon this remedy for rheumatic pains. If the pains have a burning, this remedy generally does not give good response. The 200th potency acts well when given with warm water. In biochemic therapy, this remedy is given in 6x potency with warm water and it acts far better.

Modalities: Pains are worse on touch, in night, by cold, on right side and cold bathing. Pains are better by warmth, bending double, friction and pressure.

MEDORRHINUM

It is a valuable remedy for chronic and obstinate type of pains in all the three, rheumatism, gout and arthritis and has a special action when the well-selected remedies fail to bring relief. It is a powerful and deep acting nosode for sycotic constitutions and has a relation with spinal and nervous diseases. It can be given as an intercurrent remedy when the symptoms agree. There is a pain in the whole length of spine and the back is sore to touch. A burning heat extends from nape of neck to spine. The neck has stiffness and pains in thunderstorm.

Modalities: Pain is worse when one thinks of ailments, from heat and patient feels better at sea shore, in damp weather, from fresh air and lying on abdomen.

NUX VOMICA

Nux vomica is specially indicated for torticollis (wry neck). Wry neck with shooting pain and stiffness in the nape of neck either from nervous shock or cold is the symptom for this remedy. The pains are aggravated in the morning. There is also bruised type of pain and pulling sensation in the neck and below scapulae. Neuralgia is present in cervico-brachial region, which is worse by touching. The pains are more on right shoulder and deltoid.

PHYTOLLACA DECANDRA

This remedy is particularly good for glandular affections. Its action is on periosteum, fibrous and osseous tissues, fascie and muscles sheaths have shooting and lancinating pains. Pains come and go suddenly in this remedy and they wander from place to place. Right side of neck is stiff. Best suited to persons having syphilitic miasm.

Modalities: Pains are worse in the morning when rising, wetting, exposure to rains and dampness, in the night, by pressure and more on right side of neck. Drinking hot liquids and warm applications aggravate the pains. Pains better in summer, by rest and in dry weather.

PARIS QUADRIFOLIA

Head symptoms of this remedy are marked and verified

(Boericke) and this must be verified when giving this remedy. Aches in the head as from pulling a string from eyes to occiput. Neck symptoms are weight and weariness in the nape of neck and across shoulders. Neuralgia, beginning in left intercostals region and extending into left arm, which become stiff and fingers feel numb. Tension and weakness is felt in the muscles of neck and nape. Sensation as if neck were stiff and swollen on turning it and on stooping, a weight is felt in the neck.

Modalities: Pains are more on touching, by motion and excessive thinking. Open air also aggravates the pains. The pains are less by rest taking.

RHUS TOX

This remedy is widely used by Homoeopaths for skin, rheumatic pains, mucous membrane affections and typhoid type of fevers. Pains are tearing type spread over a large surface of nape of neck, loins and extremities. There is also stiffness in the neck with rigidity and paralytic weakness of joints.

Modalities: These are to be observed in strict compliance, if Rhus tox is selected. The pains are worse during sleep, cold, wet weather and after rains. It is mostly in night and prefers right side or lying on the back. Pains are felt more when first moving after rest and after storms. The pains are better by warm dry weather, by motion, walking, and change of position, rubbing, on warm applications and from stretching out limbs.

RHODODENDRON

The true guiding symptom of this remedy is pain in the neck worse before a storm and rheumatism in hot season. Pains are in bones of neck in spots. The neck is stiff and has rigidity. There is rheumatic tension and drawing in muscles of nape of neck with sensation as if the pains are going from within to outwards. Some times pains radiate to dorsal regions or head, mostly the descending pains.

Modalities: The pains are worse before a storm and all symptoms reappear in rough weather. They are mostly in the night or early morning. The pains are better after the storm breaks, by eating and by warmth.

STRYCHNINUM

Sharp pain in the neck extending down to spine. The neck is stiff and painful especially on the left side. The pains are of gnawing, cramping, electric-like and agonizing nature. A sense of rigidity is felt in the cervical region. Cramping pains are felt suddenly in the neck and then they return at intervals. Intense itching in the whole of back is also felt.

Modalities: Pains are worse in the morning, by touch and noise and by motion or exertion. The pains are less when lying on back.

SPONGIA

It is a deep acting remedy in which rheumatic symptoms

are secondary to heart affections, thyroid and chest problems. Painful stiffness of the muscles of neck, especially on the left side and on turning the head to right side are major symptoms. Pains are of tensive nature and more on bending head backwards. There is a cracking in the neck on stooping and cracking pain is felt close to left scapula.

SULPHUR

The king of anti-psoric, Sulphur has an important role in the treatment of rheumatic and arthritic complaints. Its chief symptom is painful stiffness with or without effusion. Neck symptoms are stiffness in the nape with paralytic sprained pain. There is also a cracking sound in the vertebrae of neck when the neck is moved, especially bending the neck forward. Sulphur has a chief symptom of burning. If there is tension and burning in nape of neck or between the scapulae when moving the head, sulphur is not to be forgotten. With neck pains, if skin ailments accompany, the remedy can be granted as acting more to the benefit of patient.

Modalities: Pains are worse when standing, at rest, at night, warmth of bed, washing, bathing, in the morning by 11 AM, evening, from alcoholic stimulants and periodically. Pains are better when lying on right side, from drawing up affected limbs and dry warm weather.

THUJA

This is anti-sycotic remedy and does not play a vital role in rheumatic or arthritic complaints. If the other symptoms are in order with the remedy, this remedy can be used for cervical spondylosis. There is uneasiness in the nape of neck initially and the onset is insidious. Tension on the skin of nape when moving the head and cracking sound in cervical vertebrae on moving the head are two chief symptoms. In some cases, a burning sensation is also felt and pains go on shifting from one side to another although it is more beneficial for left-sided manifestations. There is more of sweating on the uncovered parts or all over except the head. Early morning diarrhea is also one symptom of this remedy.

Modalities: Pains are worse in night, during rest, from the heat of bed, at 3 a.m. or 3 p.m., from cold damp air, after breakfast, after taking fats or coffee, complaint after vaccination and on left side every alternate day. Pains are better by gentle rubbing, on motion of neck, in the open air, perspiration, wrapping up neck and head and when drawing the limbs.

CHAPTER 12

THERAPEUTIC SUGGESTIONS

VIEWS OF DIFFERENT AUTHORS

In the earlier chapter general therapeutic suggestions have been given but it will be of more value if the readers, in respect of cervical spondylosis, know the views of prominent authors. I have tried to focus on few remedies and not all, so that there is no confusion. At the end of this chapters we shall try to summarize the remedies mostly used.

1. DR. R.B.BISHAMBHAR DAS IN BOOK 'SELECT YOUR REMEDY'

ACTAEA SPICATA

Pain in the neck with right arm lame feeling, paralytic weakness and pain in hands and palms very sensitive to pressure are the chief symptoms of this remedy.

CALCAREA FLUOR

Indurated cervical glands, calcareous deposits, stony hardness, synovial swelling, vertigo, lumbago, cracking in joints, sensitive to cold damp weather, worse during rest and better by heat are the symptoms.

CAUSTICUM

The remedy is useful when there is swelling of cervical glands, stiffness of neck, pain in shoulder blades, arms and hands and paralytic feeling in right hand.

CAULOPHYLLIUM

Stiffness of neck, pulling in sterno-cleidomastoid drawing head to left, fingers stiff and drawing and cutting pain when closing hands are the symptoms of this remedy.

FLUORIC ACID

Stiffness and pain in the neck, weakness, lameness and numbness of forearm and neck, pricking pain in fingers, difficulty in writing, stitching in hip bones and soles of feet are the indications for use of this remedy.

GNAPHALIUM

Giddy feelings on rising up, numbness of limbs alternating with neck pains, which are of cutting type, are some of the symptoms.

LEDUM

Tearing pain in neck and shoulders, hands, arms and on raising arms, stinging in hands, tearing in arms and numbness of arms are some of the indications.

RHODODENDRON

Tension and drawing in muscles of nape of neck, stiff neck, rigidity of neck with tearing in shoulders are the symptoms of this remedy.

2. DR. T.P. CHATTERJEE IN HIS BOOK, 'TIT BITS OF HOMOEOPATHY'.

CERVICAL SPONDYLOSIS

Euphrasia is useful for slipped disc and spondylosis. This remedy has pain worse on exertion, bending and stooping.

Tellurium is almost specific. Use 30th potency twice so long as improvement is there. If it stops working or condition deteriorates, use 1M potency.

When single vertebra is sensitive to touch, three doses of *Agaricus* 1M given for a day will cure.

Spondylosis with vertigo and nausea, *Theridion* is the remedy.

Numbing pains coming and going slowly, extending from neck to right arm and hands are the symptoms for *Platina* 30 to 1M.

For characteristic pain in first vertebra, *Nux vomica* is the remedy.

Neck pain only when neck is moved, the remedy is *Aurum muriaticum natronatum*. (Reference of Dr. Shankaran given by Dr. Chatterjee).

Aggravation in cold damp weather, the remedy is *Dulcamara 200*, which should be given one dose daily for four consecutive days.

Dr. Chatterjee also states about *management of rheumatic cervical spondylosis*. He advises bed rest during pains, avoiding rich food, applying hot fomentation, doing light exercise and light work, walking should be tolerable, and supporting collar to be worn for prevention of pains. Diet should contain proteins, fruits, vegetables and starches, saccharin be avoided. No liquor, fish and eggs should be allowed. There should be no mental stress and strain. For women, he says that women should not lift weight more than 12 kg and men should not carry weights more than half of their body weight.

DR. T.P.CHATTERJEE IN HIS BOOK, 'HIGHLIGHTS OF HOMOEOPATHIC PRACTICE'.

CERVICAL SPONDYLOSIS

In chronic stage when pain is worse in cold and wet weather. *Dulcamara* 1M, 10 M.

Reduced inter-vertebral spaces in cervical region with presence of osteophytes, pain in night, pain in forearms all the time, paroxysmal numbness in hand with pain in upper arm when lying on it, the remedy is *Natrium mur* 1M.

When patient likes warm bath and is relieved by it, the medicine is *Carbo animalis* 1M.

In right-sided shooting pain in the neck, use *Kalmia* 30.

When the cause of the pain is injury, give *Arnica* 1M.

CERVICALGIA

Nux vomica, Silicea and Rhus tox are three main remedies. *Nux vomica* is to be given in 12th potency and the higher potency will aggravate.

3. DR. K.P.S.DHAMA AND DR. SUMAN DHAMA IN BOOK, 'HOMOEOPATHY: THE COMPLETE HANDBOOK'.

CERVICAL SPONDYLOSIS

Vertigo, worse closing eyes due to degeneration of spinal cord, *Theridion* 30, four hourly.

With muscular weakness, perspiration of hands, especially in bachelors, *Conium* 200 or 1M, 3 hourly 3 doses.

With numbness worse night, *Kali iodide* 200 or 1M, 3 hourly, 3 doses.

Head remedy, tearing pains with weakness, *Acid phos* 30, four hourly.

Pain nape of neck, better movement, worse rest, cold and damp, after icy cold water, *Rhus tox* 200 or 1M, four hourly, and three doses.

Pain in neck, back and limbs after exposure to dry cold winds, better from heat and least movement, great thirst- *Bryonia* 200, 3 hourly, three doses.

Shooting pain in the neck, shoulders 'crack' on movement, legs heavy daytime and ache at night, *Pulsatilla* 200, 3 doses, 3 hourly.

4. DR. J.N.SHINGHAL IN HIS BOOK, 'BEDSIDE PRESCRIBER'.

ACUTE CASES OF STIFF NECK

Stiff neck due to draught or chill, pains worse on moving the head, the remedy is *Aconite* 30, 1 hourly.

Stiff neck from damp and cold, pain after lying with head in uncomfortable position, the remedy is *Dulcamara* 30, one hourly.

Stiff neck as if sprained, head twisted to one side and the medicine is *Lachnantes*.

Stiff neck, head and neck retracted, rheumatic pains, the medicine is *Actaea racemosa*.

5. DR. N.C.GHOSH IN HIS BOOK, 'COMPARATIVE MATERIA MEDICA.'

STIFF NECK

Stiffness with head and neck pulled to one side, the remedy is *Lachnantes tincture*.

Stiffness with gouty pain in neck, cannot move the neck. Pain in shoulders when lowering the scapula, the medicine is *Anacardium*.

Stiffness and pain in neck, which is reduced when moving the neck slowly, use *Pulsatilla*.

Stiffness and pain in neck, which is reduced when moving the neck vigorously, use *Conium*.

6. DR. CONSTANTINE HERRING IN HIS BOOK, 'DOMESTIC PHYSICIAN'.

WRY NECK

It is a pain with rheumatic affection of neck. It is generally occasioned by exposures to a draught of air or by turning the head suddenly around. *Aconite* or *Belladona* may bring a cure. Should these be insufficient, Cocculus, *Rhus tox* or *Bryonia* will mostly suffice.

7. DR. K.C. BHANJA IN HIS BOOK, 'HOMOEOPATHIC PRESCRIBER'.

STIFF NECK

Stiffness with violent pain in upper three dorsal vertebrae extending through scapulae, the remedy is *Kalmia*.

Stiffness with aching and bruised pain in the neck and between scapulae, *Rhus tox* will cure.

Stiffness of whole spine, the medicine is *Agaricus*.

Stiffness from neck to small of back and sacrum with intolerable pain on slightest motion or turning, pain not noticed on touch or during rest, the remedy is *Guaiacum*.

8. DR. A.C.DUTTA IN HIS BOOK, 'SNAPSHOT PRESCRIBER'.

NECK

Pain drawing with stiffness, *Cyclamen*.

Pain extending down to left hand, *Kalmia.*

Pain in the nape of neck, *Acid phos.*

Pain stabbing in the neck, *Kali bromatum.*

STIFFNESS

And painful on motion-	*Tarentula*
After taking cold-	*Ferrum phos*
Due to damp sheet	*Rhus tox*
Glands swollen with	*Mercurius solubilis*
Head drawn back	*Actaea racemosa*
Head drawn to one side	Caulophyllum
Of rheumatic origin	*Rhus tox*

9. DR. W.IDE PIERCE IN HIS BOOK 'PLAIN TALKS ON MATERIA MEDICA'.

STIFFNESS

From cold, worse right side	*Causticum* and *Belladona*
From any draft	*Calcarea phos*
Worse left side	*Actaea racemosa*
With head drawn to one sid	*Nux vomica*

10. DR.JOHN H. CLARKE IN HIS BOOK 'PRESCRIBER'.

STIFFNESS

Due to exposure to cold, lower part tearing pain, movement aggravation and pain extending to shoulders

Aconite 3

Neck bent to one side *Actaea racemosa* 3

Pulling of neck, bent head *Antim tart*

Stiff neck, spraining on movement, bending neck to one side

Lachesis Q

With pain, aggravation on touch and movement

Bryonia

Paralysis of neck *Colchicum* 3

Due to cold and dampness, pain more on lying on

occiputal position *Dulcamara* 3

Dry cold winds, storms reason for pain in neck

Rhododendron 3

Pain on right side *Chelidonium* 1

Note: Stiff neck should be given hot fomentation and then wrapping should be done.

SUMMARY OF THE REMEDIES PREFERRED
BY THE ABOVE MENTIONED TEN AUTHORS

Above-mentioned ten authors have suggested a total of forty remedies. These remedies have been indicated on different symptoms and cannot be made comparable for reaching the most benefiting remedies. Every remedy has its own sphere of symptoms.

Two authors have preferred Agaricus, Theridion, Acid phos, Pulsatilla, Lachnanthes, Rhododendron, Nux vomica, Conium and Aconite. These means nine out of forty remedies are more useful provided the symptoms agree. **Marks 2/40**

Three authors out of forty remedies have preferred Kalmia, Dulcamara and Bryonia. **Marks 3/40**

Four authors out of forty remedies have preferred Actaea racemosa. **Marks 4/40**

Five authors have preferred Rhus tox. **Marks 5/40**

We can draw a conclusion now:

Rhus tox is the **first** remedy to be thought over for cervical spondylosis.

The **second** remedy is **Actaea racemosa.**

The **third remedies in the row** are **Bryonia, Dulcamara** and **Kalmia.**

It must be kept in mind that the above remedies have to be given basing upon the totality of symptoms. This calculation is just a summary of the views of great authors.

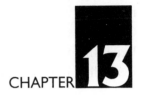

REPERTORY SUGGESTIONS

THE REMEDIES shown in this section pertain to cervical spondylosis. In selecting a remedy, the totality of the symptoms of the disease has to be viewed.

COMMON MEDICINES FOR CERVICAL SPONDYLOSIS

Arn., arg-m., bell., bar-c., calc-p., caust., cimi., cocc., colch., dulc., kali-i., lach., lyc., med., mur-ac., nat-s., nit-ac., nux-v., pet., ph-ac., rad., rut., sec., spong., stan., sul., ver-a.

CERVICAL REGION

Coldness
Morning	Ran-s.
Evening	Spong., dulc.
Creeping	Sil.
Extending to occiput	Chel.
Extending to sacrum, on lying	Thuj.

Constriction
Agar., apis, asar., bell., chel., dulc., glon., lach., nux-m., sep.

Cracking
Bending head backward	Sulph.
Rising from stooping, on	Nicc.
Stooping, on	Spong.
Swallowing aggravate	Thuj.

Formication
Arund., carl., dulc., lac-c., phos., sabin., sec., spong.

Heat
Afternoon	Con.
Afternoon, cold hands with	Sumb.
Afternoon, 7 to 8 PM	Fl-ac.

Heaviness
Morning	Nux-v.
Walking after	Rhus-t.
Weight upon	Coloc., Nux-v., Kali-c., Par., Phos., Rhus-t., tub.

Pain

Right	Graph., sulph.
Left	Con., can., carb-an., thuj.
Right to left	Calc-p.
Right to left on turning head	Cinnb., graph., mez.
Rising morning amel.	Alum.
Forenoon	Agar., stry.
Afternoon	Calc-p., chel., chin-s.,
4 p.m.	mag-p., nux-v., thuj.
	Chin-s
Going to bed	Alum.
Looking up	Form.
Midnight	Lach., mag-s.
Draft of air	Rhus-t., calc-p., cimic.
Fresh air amel.	Psor.
Alternating with headache	Hyos.
Ascending	Ph-ac.
Blowing nose	Kali-bi.
Breathing deeply	Chel.
Bending head forward amel.	Gels., sanic., laur.
Bending head forward on	Cimic., graph., stann.
Bending head backward	Bell., chel., cic., cinnb., cycl., kali-c., laur., lyc., valer.
Bending head backward amel.	Cycl., lac-c., lyss., syph.
Bending head left to	Par.
Bending head right to	Sulph.
Chewing aggravate	Zinc.
Coughing on	Alum., bell., caps., sulph.
Eating after	Nux-v.
Looking up, on	Graph.
Lying on back	Graph., spig.

Lying on sides	Graph.
Lying on right side	Ferr.
Manual exertion	Ant-c.
Mental exertion	Par.
Menses, before	Nat-c., nux-v., sulph.
Menses, during	Calc., mag-c.
Motion amel.	Aur-m-n., spig.
Moving head to either side	Agar.
Rising arm, on	Ant-c., graph.
Reading, while	Nat-c.
Riding in carriage	Form.
Sneezing, when	Am-m., arn., mag-c.
Standing in one position	Cham.
Swallowing, when	Calc-p., nat-c.
Talking from	Arn., calc., sulph.
Touch from	Chin., nux-v.
Stool after, amel.	Asaf.
Turning head to left	Alum., ant-c.
Writing, while	Carb-an., zinc.
Yawning, on	Arn., nat-s.

Pain cervical, extending to

Arms and fingers	Kalm., nux-v., par.
Arms	Nat-m., nux-v.
Arm, left	Kalm., lach., par.
Clavicles, to	Gels., nat-s
Ears, to	Bor., calc-p., cann-s., colch., lyss., thuj.
Eyes, to	Gel., lach., ph-ac., pic-ac., sel., sil.
Forehead, to	Mez., rat., sars.
Head, to	Apis., carb-v., ferr., par., pul., sil.

Occiput, to	Calc-p., chel., cinnb., dulc., eup-perf., ferr., gels., glon., kali-c., kalm., nat-c., nat-s., nat-m., phyt., sil.
Shoulders, between	Am-m., apis.
Shoulder, right	Acon., alum., lyc., phos.
Shoulder, left	Bor., bry., ran-b.
Stannum, to	Kali-bi.

Stiffness, cervical region

Eating, after	Nux-v
Lifting, from	Calc., lyc., rhus-t., sep.
Lying on back	Spig.
Menses, during	Calc.
Motion amel.	Alum., caps., ph-ac.
Rest, during	Ph-ac., rat., rhod., rhus-t.
Sleep, during	Alum.
Stool, after	Puls.
Stooping	Calc.
Turning head on	Alum., am-c., am-m., aur., bell., bry., calad., calc., chel., coloc., dulc., spong.
Turning head to left	Alum.
Turning head to right	Spong.
Violent motion amel.	Rat.
Walking, on	Anac., graph., kali-c., lach., manc., phys.
Walking, air, in open	Camph., lyc.
Washing, from	Dulc., rhus-t.
Yawning, on	Cocc., nat-m.

Nature of pain, cervical region

Pain, aching

Morning	Amyl-n., thuj.
Rising	Calc., caust.
Waking, on	Ars.
Forenoon	Agar.
Evening	Alum., zinc.
Bending head backward amel.	Cycl., lac-c.
Coughing, on	Bell.
Extending to arm	Plect.
Extending to head and shoulders	Dios.
Extending to occiputal region	Amyl-n
Extending to spine	Hell.
Extending to shoulders	Verat-v
Extending to back on going to stool	Verat.

Pain, boring

Bar-c., mag-p., psor., sulph., Eating, after aggravation	Sulph.

Pain, burning

Morning	Am-c
Afternoon	Fago.
Evening	Mag-c.
Itching, tickling	Calc.
Moving head agg.	Nat-s., plb.
Paroxysms	Plb.
Piercing	Apis
Scratching, after	Mag-c.
Sleep amel.	Calc.
Spots, in	Kali-br.

Stinging	Glon.
Swallowing	Petr.
Touched, when	Nat-m.
Extending to clavicle	Nat-s.
Extending to down back	Med.
Extending to occiput	Calc.

Pain, cramp like

Evening	Mang.
Eating, after	Sep.
Moving head	Cimic., mang.
Sneezing	Arn.
Swallowing, when	Zinc.
Yawning	Arn.

Pain, cutting

Ang., berb., canth., dig., eup.per., glon., graph., grat., kali-b., naja., samb., stry., thuj.

Pain, dragging Gels., pic-ac.

Pain, drawing

Right	Nux-v., sulph., zinc.
Morning	Ant-c., cimic., nux-v., staph.
Morning, bending head forward on	Cimic.
Waking, on	Aloe., alum.
Afternoon	Calc-p., mag-c., nux-v., thuj.
Evening	Ant-c.; nat-m., thuj.
Bending head backward	Cycl., dig., valer.
Cold, damp air	Nux-m

Intermittent	Spig.
Manual exertion agg.	Ant-c.
Menses, before	Nat-c., nux-v.
Moving amel.	Alum.
Moving head agg.	Nat-c.
Reading, while	Nat-c.
Rheumatic	Anac., bor., sep., staph.
Sitting, while	Ant-c., Aur-m, nux-v..
Stooping, on	Ant-c.,berb., canth., rhus-t.
Turning head	Ant-c., chel., hyos.
Turning head to left	Ant-c.
Extending to ear	Cann-s., colch.
Extending to elbow	Lyc.
Extending to head	Apis, calc., ferr., carb-v.
Extending to occiput	Am-c., asaf., chel., coloc., nat-c., nux-v., psor., rat., spong.
Extending to scapula	Ant-c.
Extending to shoulders	Chel., con., kali-n., lyc., phyt., camph., bor.
Extending to left shoulder and scapula while walking in open air	Bor.
Extending upwards	Ambr., calc., cann-s., petr.

Pain, gnawing   Nat-s., thuj.

Pain, lancinating   Bell., canth., claps.

Pain, pressing

Weight, as from	Anac., caps., coloc., par.
Weight, walking after	Rhus-t.

Extending to clavicle	Nat-s.
Extending to forehead or occiput	Chel.
Extending to head	Ambr., grat.
Extending to head, occiput	Guag., nat-c., nat-s., ph-ac.
Extending to head, shoulders	Ip.

Pain, sore

Left	Agar.
Morning after waking agg.	Arg-m., ph-ac.
Morning, rising after	Am-m.
Evening	Sep.
Bending head backwards	Bad., cic., hep.
Burning	Ph-ac.
Lying down	Lyc.
Motion, on	Am-m., asar., nux-v.
Motion amel.	Sulph.
Moving head	Kali-c., kalm., merc-I-f., podo.
Stooping, on	Nux-v.
Stretching, on	Nat-s.
Walking amel.	Mag-s.
Walking in open air	Sep.
Yawning	Nat-s

Pain, stitching

Morning in bed	Stann.
Afternoon	Stry.
Evening	Bov., coc-c., nat-c., thuj.
Evening, bed in	Lyc.
Night	Caust., kalm., nat-m., nat-s.

Ascending steps, on	Ph-ac.
Coughing	Alum.
Itching	Stann.
Lying, while	Caust., kali-i.
Moving, on	Alum., camph., dig., guaj., merc., sars.
Moving head	Acon., am-m., bad., dig., samb., sars.,thuj.
Moving head forward and backward	Cocc.
Pulsating	Cocc.
Sitting, while	Lyc.
Sitting, amel.	Tarax.
Sitting, bent over	Sulph.
Sneezing, on	Am-m., lyc., mag-c.
Standing	Tarax.
Stinging	Apis., bar-c., calc., lyss., phyt.
Stooping, on	Agar., sulph.
Stretching out amel.	Sulph.
Swallowing amel.	Spong.
Talking, while	Calc.
Turning head, on	Alum., verat.
Walking, on	Ph-ac.
Extending to ear	Bov., stry., thuj.
Extending to eye	Sel.
Extending to head	Kalm.
Extending to lumbar region	Stry., tep.
Extending to occiput	Kali-c., ph-ac.
Extending to sacrum	Lyc., stry.
Extending to shoulders	Am-m., laur., stry., thuj.
Extending to right shoulder	Alum.

Extending upwards	Berb., lyc.
Extending to vertex	Rhus-t., sil.
Extending between cervical and first dorsal vertebra	Staph.
Pain, tearing	
Left	Rat., sulph.
Morning	Kali-c.,Stram.
Afternoon	Mag-c.
Evening	Nux-v.
Night	Rhod.
Midnight, before, waking on	Sulph.
Chill, during	Ars-h
Coughing	Alum.
Jerking	Aur., caps., rat.
Lying, while	Lyc.
Menses, during	Am-m., mag-c.
Motion, on	Carb-v., dig., ign., kali-bi., verat.
Motion of head	Am-m., canth., nat-c., sulph.
Paroxysmal	Nux-v.
Pressure amel.	Zinc.
Sneezing	Am-m.
Stool, after amel.	Asaf.
Sudden	Nat-c.
Walking, while	Rat.
Warm room, in	Caust.
Extending down back	Mag-c., rhod.
Extending to ear	Thuj.
Extending to forehead	Rat., sars.
Extending to vertex	Rat.
Extending to shoulders	Alum., am-m., thuj., til.

Extending to right shoulder in evening after lying down	Lyc.
Extending to either side to top of head	Lach.
Extending upwards	Berb., canth., lach.
Extending to spine	Lach.
Extending to spine at night	Caust.

Pain, pulsating

Holding head backward amel.	Lyss., manc.
Lying down, on	Plb.
Menses, before	Nit-ac.
Menses, during	Nit-ac., verat-v
Motion agg.	Ferr.
Raising head, stooping from	Kali-n
Sitting, while	Calc-p.
Writing agg.	Manc.
Extending to forehead and on moving or stooping	Ter.
Extending to forehead and occiput	Chel.
Extending to lumbar region	Cur.
Extending to shoulders	Apis., con.
Extending to vertebra	Kali-n.

Pain, pricking

Carb-an.

CHAPTER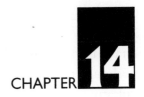

NOSODES AND SARCODES

Spondylosis, ankylosing	*Carc.
Cracking sound from turning head	Lac-hum.
Cracking sound from turning head, cervical	Syph.
Cracking sound from turning head, occiputal	Syph.
General pain, cervical	Cortico., lac-c., lyss., hyp-p., ust., pneum., syph., malaria, v-a-b., veriol.
Side, left	X-ray
Side, right	Carc., lac-hum.

Pains, nature of

Boring	Psor.
Burning	Lyss.
Cramping	Med., x-ray.
Drawing	Med.
Drawing extending to shoulders	Psor.
Pulsating	Med.
Stinging	Lyss.
Stitching, lancinating	Lyss., psor.
Tearing	Lyss., psor.
Tearing, shoulder left	Ambr.
Tearing, shoulder right	Ambr.
Wandering	Lac-c.
Tiredness, cervical neck	Malaria.

Stiffness

Cervical	Bac-7, lac-c., lac-hum., lyss., morg-g., psor., tub., variol.
Side, left	X-ray.
Side, right	Lyss., x-ray.

* Full names of above remedies

Carc.	Carcinosin
Lac-hum	Lac humanum
Syph.	Syphillinum
Cortico	Corticotrophin
Lac-c	Lac caninum
Lyss.	Lyssin (hydrophobinum)
Hyp-p	Hypophysis posterium
Ust.	Ustilago

Pneum.	Pneumococcine
Malaria	Malaria officinalis
V-a-b	Vaccine, bilie calmette guerin (BCG)
Variol.	Variolinum
X-ray	X-ray
Psor.	Psorinum
Med.	Medorrhinum
Ambr.	Ambra grisea
Bac-7	Bacillus no. 7 (paterson)
Morg-g	Morgan-gaertner
Tub.	Tuberculinum bovinum

3

PART

PART 3

CHAPTER 15

OTHER THERAPIES

TOUCH THERAPY AND CERVICAL SPONDYLOSIS

B ROADLY SPEAKING, there are three main methods of application of medicines. Removing and killing the cause of diseases by medicine is the first method called 'preventive'. Example is initial vaccinations to the infants and taking precautions in diet-intake. Ayurveda also comes in this category to some extent. People take 'Chayvan Prash' (a tonic) as preventive to coughs. The second method is the conventional system of medicines in which cure is by application of 'opposites'. This is allopathy. Example is taking of laxatives when there is constipation. The third method is 'similimum' or Homoeopathy in which cure is through such medicines, which can excite similar symptoms in a healthy body. There is no fourth primary method. All other existing methods are complementary to these three methods. They are alternatives and enhance the action of the basic three methods.

Lot of experimentation or hit and trial has been made with medicines of Homoeopathy. The doctrine of single remedy, the classical way, combination with biochemic medicines and patent mixtures are few examples. Homoeopathy is being amalgamated with naturopathy, magneto therapy, acupressure, acupuncture, Shiatsu and astrology to work as complementary to homoeopathy. If you believe that doctor's first aim is to cure the patient, all complimentary therapies should be acceptable provided these do not disturb the action of basic homoeopathic medicines. Those who want to reap better results and insert novelty in treatment, 'touch therapy' will be highly useful, commercially or otherwise.

SHIATSU THERAPY

It is almost a parallel therapy with that of touch therapy and is called **'Shiatsu'**. Shiatsu is an old customary oriental therapy, which has its origin in China. It got relayed to Japan from China and then to the western countries. Shiatsu believes in balance and harmony of health and that the body is not separate from the mind. Body is a complete unit. The method of application of Shiatsu is somewhat similar to acupressure. Pressure on various parts of the body makes it effective. It must be kept in mind that 'touch' is an integral part of Shiatsu through which positive energy of the doctor is relayed to the patient. Shiatsu has been mentioned here for the purpose of knowledge of readers and its only relevance under the reference is 'touch'. We revert back to our subject now.

IMPORTANCE OF 'TOUCH'?

Touch therapy is beyond any other conventional methods of treatments. Touching the patients through skilled methods, explained at the end of this topic, can make a difference to the benefit of patients. Here is a historical explanation of touch therapy:

- Touching each other is as ancient as the birth of mankind. A man without a touch with society is an animal.

- Embracing and kissing are varieties of touch between genders emitting heaven pleasures. The 'give and take' of sex is finer mode of touch-doctrine.

- Hugging friends and relatives relieve tensions, improve relations and bring nearness.

- Crying babies, when hugged by mothers, stop weeping and feel secured by the touch of mothers.

- Patting on the backs of youngsters by elders is a magic of touch that boosts good deeds.

- Physiotherapy, osteopathy and chiropractic are practical acts of touch giving fruitful results.

- Blessings on the heads of children by elders or touching the feet of elders are acts of touch that dignify and moralize them, respectively.

- Give a pat on the head of a dog and it will react majestically by waving its tail and this graceful expression is a miracle of touch.

- The patient feels satisfied and cared for when the doctor

touches his pulse and examines by instruments. It is a fact that doctors who do not touch their patients through instruments or otherwise are not popular.

Indians have traditional and cultural affinity with touch and miraculous cures have been witnessed in the past with touch-blessings of great saints. When Swami Ramakrishna touched the forehead of Swami Vivekananda, (a non-believer in God, initially) he experienced the mystic joy of God's existence. This touch changed the course of his life. Touch is a powerful weapon. Touch of fingers compel computers obey, enable machines roar and fly, control infinite functions with remotes and make every possible fiction or function a reality. Nothing in the world can be done without the help of touch. If this 'touch' is put into practice by some effective methods of healing, it can do wonders. This possibility cannot be denied. Here is a rational study.

RELATION WITH HOMOEOPATHY

Touch therapy has not been given importance in Homoeopathy. If you study the sermons of S. Hahnemann, the father of Homoeopathy (aphorism 83 to 104 of his book 'Organon'), you will be surprised that there are no specific instructions to check the patients physically. Under the footnote of aphor. 104, Hahnemann shows his dislike for allopathy and he does not want to imitate allopathy in any way. He criticizes allopaths for hurried examination like feeling pulse and looking at the tongue. This appears to be the reason that Hahnemann never formulated any Materia Medica of the kind where medicines could be given according to results of values and outcome of laboratory tests. He rates upon symptoms mainly. The reason was probably non availability of laboratory tests for blood, urine etc. The results of such tests also amount to symptoms and there was no reason why a brilliant scholar like Hahnemann could not have accomplished formulation of a Materia Medica according to results of tests.

A general, peculiar, mental, emotional, subjective, objective and concomitant symptom derived from interrogation of patients and his relatives is the main principle of Homoeopathic theory. On the other hand, Hahnemann did not emphasize much upon physical examination of the patient and hence 'touch' did not come to his attention. In the modern education system of Homoeopathy, the methods of diagnosis (Thermometer, pulse rate, stethoscope, blood pressure measuring instrument and numerous pathological tests) have changed to an extent that homoeopathy is now at par with that of conventional system. This is a good sign although it is a deviation from the main principle of homoeopathic culture. With advent of times, every good change has to be adopted be it from any system. Use of these diagnostic gadgets and laboratory tests give opportunity of touch to the doctor. Leave aside the benefits of these gadgets; this at least strengthens the touch-theory that is being discussed.

What remains pertinent with homoeopathy is that Hahnemann emphasized on the existence of vital force in our body. A force that is not located in any organ of the body and it still exists. He states that without the assistance of active remedies of human art, the vital force cannot overcome even the slight acute diseases. By human art, he means help of homoeopathic medicines. He is very clear about principle of organic vital force. It opposes only a weak resistance to the invading morbific enemy. When the disease grows, it opposes a greater resistance but at best it is only an equal resistance. If the patient is weak, the vital force is not even equal but weaker. The vital force is neither capable, nor destined, nor created for over-powering resistance. (Reference- chronic diseases by Hahnemann)

So, it can be concluded that without the assistance of energy medicine or energy itself, vital force cannot overcome disease. Hahnemann leaves no doubt that vital force has definite relation with the body. How can it be visualized or seen in some other form? How? It is another question.

We know that life started from a minute cell. It got its physical components in nine months but at some junction, a force or life or living animation entered the cell or organism either at the time of conception, during the changes in its shape or after the conception. This 'live' being remains in the body till death. Naturally when it leaves the body, death occurs. During its whole spell of residence in the body, the 'live' undergoes fluctuations and the body reflects this in the form of weakness, disorder and disease. So the impact of condition of 'live' has a mirror that shows the physical condition of body. During the avenues of fluctuations, if body is strengthened with some additional energy, the 'live' may get restored to 'near' normal, if not absolute normal. In homoeopathy, it is done by energy medicines but here physical aspect is missing altogether. We have physiotherapist, osteopaths, chiropractic practitioners, manipulators and the massagers to effect physical aspect of strengthening the body. Beauty saloons are also doing the same job. Whatever benefit is experienced with the help of these agents, this is result of 'touch' and enhance energy of body. But these measures do partial work and this is sufficient in its own sphere, even if it is partial.

THE EXPLANATION OF TOUCH THERAPY

You will agree that everyone has a systematic electrical or magnetic potential within the body. Forget about homoeopathic vital force now, which we have discussed above. There are recorded evidences of electromagnetic fields associated with human body. There was a person in Haryana whose touch sent electrical shocks to others. This was a news item in a local paper some ten years back. It may not be authenticated but the case of a 19-year-old girl in Ontario, Canada is recorded. After a short illness, she could pick a pen with her open palm by the power of electromagnetic properties. This was in 1879. In 1895 at Missouri, a fourteen-year-old girl turned into an electrical dynamo. When reaching for metal objects, her finger tips gave sparks of high voltage. (Courtesy: page 62 - Book 'Science of Homoeopathy' by George Vithoulkas)

This sort of potential exhibits an invisible electro-dynamic field around our body. This field is not only in possession of human beings but it is with all living and non-living objects. 'Kirlian photography', the latest camera to picture aura, establishes all this. Every object has its fluctuating field of energy around its shape. We can call it 'aura'. Aura is not a new term for Indians. Basing upon fantastical fictions loaded with magical self-experienced facts and mythological conceptions achieved through ancient holy books of our culture (Vedas and Puranas), aura is near to reality. Painters and creative scholars in the ancient past have visualized pictures of Gods depicting a glowing light behind their heads. This is aura. According to the belief, if aura of a person is strong, he is supposed to be healthy. Another belief is that who so ever comes in contact with high-aura-possessed persons, he is electrified mentally and influenced physically. We have examples of many great saints and Gurus of modern times (Osho, Sai Baba, Asa Ram ji, Sudhanshu ji, Anandmayi Maa and others) who attract thousands of people with their glory, excellent oratory and personality. Even many cults have started in their names. We see them, become their disciples and listen to them on television shows everyday. Thousands of their books are published and video/audio tapes are sold. What is all this? Is it not a potential being relayed by them and does it not tranquilize the listeners? I am not particularly exhibiting a religious insight, though most religious traditions owe their survival to the basic fact, the spiritualism. Most of history and human societies have thought their first duty to hand over what they have learnt. Truth is always eternal and some novel ways of life are always under discovery. Touch therapy is an attempt to resolve dilemmas of health by imparting specific doctrine in a novel way, the eternal and the acquired.

If a person with strong aura touches a person with weak aura, the *law of conduction* has to take place. Flow of energy from hot to cold and from strong to weak is inevitable. No one can deny this fact. There is an old saying that those who believe in goodness, expect goodness from others, promote goodness to benefit others and deliver abundance of goodness by their good deeds or verdicts, are real saints. Compare them with doctors. Doctors possess three of the above qualities explained on goodness. No doctor is disbelieved when he says that the patient is 'out of danger' after he returns from the operation theatre and after doing a surgery. He is definitely relied upon. Doctors possess a high potential aura and during an operation, a doctor is capable of relaying his potential to the patient through invisible vibrations, oscillation and waves of his skilled hands and instruments. In other words this job is accomplished by means of touch. *Surgery is the highest mode of touch therapy.*

EXPERIENCE THE MAGIC OF TOUCH

Now is the turn of an experiment. Do it yourself to believe it. Point the tip of your right index finger towards the center of your forehead (in between your eyebrows). Keep a slight air gap between the tip of finger and forehead skin for some seconds. Now touch the tip of finger with the forehead so gently that it is like a feather-touch. You will feel a mystic sensation of flow of energy. If you conduct this act on the forehead of other person, he or she may feel headache till the time your finger remains pointing to the forehead. In the same fashion if you feather-touch your temples, closed eyelids, center of nape of neck above cervical vertebrae, soles of feet and central area below the lower lip (above chin), you will feel the flow of energy. These are energy points where from relay of energy is possible. This is felt both by receiver and giver.

RELAY YOUR ENERGY TO THE NEEDY

The most practical energy relay station is tip of finger. *If tips of fingers of both receiver and giver are joined under the stated condition of feathery touch, the result is positive.* The touch should be between the right hand finger- tips of doctor with the right hand finger-tips of the patient. The touch should be for about 10 to 20 seconds at a time and the repetition is made four to five times.

Before practicing this therapy, a briefing to the patient is essential. You will find your selected remedies work better. Homoeopathic medicines are energy medicines and touch therapy also pertains to relay of energy. Touch therapy will act complimentary to homoeopathic remedies. It is not a claim. The conditions vary, the persons vary and the situations vary. If you are a good doctor with strong aura, it will work.

Human body is a living dynamic science and science has no borders of experimentations. The more you do, the more you gain.

One important note is that during this therapy of relay of energy, you will never be lacking in your stored energy as is in the case of blood donors.

MAGNET THERAPY

The above method of relay of your energy through tips of fingers should be first done and results seen after twelve hours. Along with this, a suitable single homoeopathic remedy should also be tried. In case this does not give enough relief, the touch by magnets can be tried. Let us have a brief knowledge of magnet therapy first.

Treatment of ailments done by touching the body with magnets for some time is called Magneto therapy. Magnet means attraction by means of physical touch. If the attraction is through mental power, this is touch therapy and if the attraction is through magnets touching, it is Magnet therapy. There flows a magnetic current in our earth. The modern science does not deny this. It is also well established by our ancestors that there is a link between the current of earth with the blood circulating veins and arteries of our body. The north pole of the earth has power to control infections of the diseases while the south pole of the earth has stored energy. Keeping the current of the earth and the body in alignment, our olden mythological books (Vedas and Puranas) suggest that our head should be in the north direction while we sleep. Upon death of a person, his or her legs are drawn towards south and his/her body is placed on floor. These Hindu traditional rites are being followed since centuries and they have definite relation with earth's magnetic power. The death of a person gets easy without much of pains in this way, is the belief. This is to bring the flow of the current of the earth in accordance with bioelectrical current of body. *Earth itself is a big magnet.* If we suspend a magnet in the air, it will turn towards north-south direction due to the influence of earth's magnetic field. Earth has two magnetic poles, south and north. A unit called 'Gauss' measures the strength of magnets. In magnet therapy, up to 1500 gauss capacity magnets are used. An instrument called gauss meter is available for measuring this. The magnet therapy has been discussed about and well established by great philosophers like Aristotle and Plato. Even the father of Homoeopathy, Dr. Hahnemann was influenced by this therapy. He used to carry a stick having magnets in his hand to examine his patients. Hahnemann was a conductor of various experiments.

It is a known fact that during sleep, our brain and heart develop strong magnetic fields. Its strength is about 3000,000 kilogauss. This strength varies from time to time. The modern scientists take the utility of this magnetic field of the body for conducting EEG and ECG tests. The biological rhythm of heart and maintaining temperature of the body are partly done by the current of this magnetic field. When there is some disease, this magnetic field gets disturbed. Our blood (RBC) has about 4 percent of iron and when a magnet is applied on the point of disturbance, the magnetic flow in the blood changes and gets re-organized and body becomes normal. When the flow of blood is normalized by this method, there will be sufficient flow of oxygen and nutritional elements in the blood. The blood cells will thus get strengthened. In some disease of heart, lungs, kidneys and liver, increase of cholesterol, calcium and urea matters. With the help of magnets, these can be dissolved. Similarly the diseases related with blood cells, pains, swellings, stiffness, bone pains and rheumatism etc. can be treated by the help of magnet application. In the tissues of the body, there are ions. More of them are in the blood. These ions act as good conductor of electricity. In the fats, bones and muscles, the quantity of ions are less and they are not good conductor of electricity. This is the reason why application of magnets is better when applied on areas where blood, arteries and veins are more in our body. It is, therefore, essential that some parts of the body are identified for application of magnets.

About 14 mediums (meridians) have been selected in whole of the body (like acupressure and acupuncture points which will be discussed in the following chapter). These are divided into 12 couplets (paired meridians) and 2 singular meridians. Every point has particular flow of magnetic field and when magnets are applied on these points, there is a positive response towards a cure. As a matter of fact, the acupuncture points is an allied science with magnet therapy and most of the magnet therapy experts use these points as the areas of application of magnets.

There are some precautions in this treatment.

- The magnet therapy should not be conducted immediately after meals. There should be at least two hours gap.

- If the patient has taken cold drinks, ice cream or any thing that is cold, this therapy should not be done. Let there be a wait for an hour or so.

- Strong power magnets should not be used on brain, heart and eyes.

- Magnets of high power should not be kept together and should also be away from watches and clocks. Magnets should be kept in their containers.

For **treatment of cervical spondylosis,** there is a need for use of strong magnets. North pole magnets should be applied on neck's right side, if the pain is on right side and south pole magnets be placed on left side of neck, if the pain is on left side. If there is extension of pains from neck to the shoulders of elbows, South Pole magnets should be placed on shoulders and elbow. Besides the above points, a point SI-3 is also to be explored and magnets be placed on it as well after an hour of placing magnets on neck and shoulders. This SI-3 point is outside the palm, about 5 cm below the base of little finger. For this point, the magnet is to be placed on the palms. Points of both the hands are to be treated by magnets.

It is better for the homoeopath to study in details about Magnet therapy. A lot of books are available with M/s B. Jain Publishers on the subject along with the gadgets for application. *Full details of magnetic equipment and books concerning magnet therapy can be had from M/s B. Jain publishers, New Delhi.*

ACCUPRESSURE THERAPY

Our body has many vulnerable points where the flow of

blood counts. These points if pressed or punctured with the help of needles normalize the flow of blood, if there is some obstruction and correct the diseases. In order to make effect on these points, a lot of therapies other than simplest pressure therapy have been developed. They are acupuncture, reflexology, shiatsu etc. but the most ancient one is acupressure. According to a saying this acupressure therapy was initiated by saints and doctors of ancient India. It was developed here and then it spread to China, Egypt, Central Asia and other countries. According to a belief, Buddhists believed in this therapy and during the spread of Buddhism, they founded the same in other countries wherever they went preaching. On the other hand, Acupuncture therapy is supposed to be initiation of China where it is said to be 5000 years old. In the olden books of China, there is mention of both acupressure and acupuncture and they claim both the therapies of their origin. Whatever may be the case, it is a fact that both the therapies are professed and practiced as a main treatment- line today in China.

It is a fact that even if mother gets headache, she will ask her children to press her head. This is the first treatment in any home even today. It is also a fact that this pressing gives instant relief to the headache, even if partial. If this example is true, there is no doubt that acupressure is born out of this technique. Birth of acupuncture has different story. There used to be fights and wars between countries during ancient times when use of arrows was one of the weapons of war. It was experienced by wounded soldiers that an arrow piercing them at some point of the body was giving them relief in respect of their old ailments of rheumatism, gout etc. This was a strange discovery of experience for doctors of the times and probably acupuncture got started.

In the olden books of China, there are about 669 points of pressure listed but the practical aspects of the therapy has shown that 90 to 100 points of the list value more and are in use for cure of diseases. In twentieth century, this art was more or less forgotten but with the leadership of Mao Tse Tung in China, this therapy got boosted and popular due to his encouragement.

Puncturing of ears and nose is a common tradition in India and this is most common in women than in men. It is a belief that these punctures meant for ornamenting the organs or for looking beautiful are beneficial for averting heart diseases. Many scholars of the therapy state that woman are not more prone to heart diseases due to this puncturing. To avoid Asthma, even now people get their ears punctured. The result was that on ear itself, doctors discovered more than 200 acupuncture points. In 1950, a Neuro-surgeon, Dr. Paul Nozier developed exclusive ear puncture therapy, which is named as 'Oracular therapy'.

The scholars and doctors of India, China and Japan believe that life is a bioelectric phenomenon. This means that our life is based upon some life-electric-current or power. This power only enable, us to move, inhales, exhale, think and enact metabolism of body. Chinese call this power as 'Chi'. In India we call it 'Pran'. This power is of two types. 'Yin' and 'Yang'. Yin is negative and Yang is positive. With the help of these negative and positive balancing, the body remains healthy. In case of any misbalance between the two, the diseases occur. These negative and positive powers flow in our blood through a special route called 'Meridian'. Chinese doctors call this as 'zing'. There are 14 major zings in our body and out of these 14, twelve zings are in couples and they are on right and left sides of the body. The rest of the two zings are in frontal central line of body and rear central line of body, vertically. Out of twelve zings, which are in couples, six are Yin meridians and other six are yang meridians. Yin meridians start from fingers of feet or from the central part of the body and extend towards fingers of hand and head. Yang meridians start from head, face or fingers of hands and extend towards earth (feet). They also start from middle of body and extend towards feet. This is the reason that every part of body is covered when we press one place or point. The only thing is to have knowledge about these points.

If you as a Homoeopath have an interest in acupressure or acupuncture, you can enquire about the concerned books from M/s B. Join Publishers, New Delhi for complete study.

CERVICAL SPONDYLOSIS TREATMENT IN ACUPRESSURE

There are only four points upon which a pressure with the help of you finger or thumb can give your relief in pain instantly.

- Behind the head (occipital) where the scalp ends and spinal joint starts, in the first central part of head, the first point occurs.

- An inch away from this central point to the left and right are two points.

- The third point is the place on the central rear area of neck where you can observe a slight raised ball. You have to press just below the bone-ball.

METHOD AND CONDITIONS OF PRESSURE APPLICATION

- The first important note is that if you have located the above points rightly, there will be pain on the points while applying pressure. This pain indicates that the points located are right. In case you experience no pain on the found out points, search for the right point nearby. You will find one.

- The second important note is that you can conduct this application of pressure at any place and at any time, you desire. It is better to do it at a place, which is quite open and where you get fresh air.

- The third important note that you can press the point with any finger but it is better if you do it with the help of your thumb, which will give more of pressure. If you still want to utilize your index finger, better place it on the nail of middle finger and press the middle finger now on the point. For easy pressure, a sort of lever called Jimmy is available in the market, which can also be purchased. Your nails should not be sharp or grown so that there is no scratch effected on the body.

- There are many methods of application of pressure. It depends upon the nature and extent of disease. These methods may be pressure by circulating the finger clock-wise around the point or anti-clockwise and pressure from sides in an angle. But the most accepted and easy is vertical pressure.

- So far as the neck pain is concerned, it is better to apply the pressure directly inside. It should be strong enough to have a feeling that something is really attacking the pain. The time for making pressure should be about 5 to 7 seconds. Now release the pressure for 5 to 7 seconds and then again press the point for 5 to 7 seconds. Repeat this pressure and gap in between for at least four times. Another easy method is to count up 13 slowly during the pressure period in your mind and release the pressure. Then again count 13 during the recess period before starting pressure again.

- In whole of the day, a total of 5 to 15 minutes should be given for this pressure in adults. For children up to the age from 3 to 12 years, the total time should be 5 to 10 minutes in a day.

- In case the patient is tired and has come from outside work, are perspiring or your heart beat is more, better allow time for rest before conducting acupressure.

- Immediately after meals, acupressure should not be conducted.

- In pregnancy, it is better not to conduct acupressure at all.

- If the patient has taken a hot or cold bath, better wait for at least one hour.

- If the patient has come back from evacuation of bowels, it is advisable to wait for half an hour.

- If you have a broken bone or injured, acupressure should not be done on the place or near the place of injury.

- In case you have taken allopathic drugs, wait for two hours before conducting acupressure.

BIBLIOGRAPHY

Organon of Medicine	*S.Hahnemann*
Chronic Diseases	*S.Hahnemann*
Lectures on Homoeopathic Materia Medica	*J.T.Kent*
Repertory of Homoeopathic Materia Medica	*J.T.Kent*
Lectures on Homoeopathic Philosophy	*J.T.Kent*
Boenninghausen's Therapeutic Pocket Book	*H.A.Robeerts*
	and *Annie C. Wilson*
Book of Surgery	*Baily and Love*
Atlas of Anatomy	*Trevor Weston*
Comparative Materia Medica and Therapeutics	*N.C.Ghosh*
Plain Talks on Materia Medica with Comparisons	*Willard Ide Pierce*
Homoeopathic Materia Medica and Repertory	*W. Boerick*
Keynotes of Leading Remedies	*H.C.Allen*
Chronic Miasms and Pseudo Psora	*J.H.Allen*
Prescriber	*John H. Clarke*
Materia Medica	*C. Herring*
Select Your Remedy	*R.B.Bishamber Das*
Homoeopathic Prescriber	*K.C.Bhanja*
Bedside Prescriber	*J.N.Shinghal*

From Old Age to Youth Through Yoga   *S. Siddhantalankar*

The Principle and Art of Cure by Homoeopathy   *H.A.Roberts*

Therapeutic Pocket Book   *Boenninghausen*

Science of Homoeopathy   *George Vithoulkas*

Homoeopathy in Cervical Spondylosis   *Farokh J.Master*

Domestic Physician   *Constantine Herring*

Repertory of Homoeopathic Nosodes and Sarcodes   *Berkley Squire*

Practice of Medicine   *F.W.Price*

Cure Aches and Pains Through Osteopathy   *Krishan Murari Modi*

Life of Hahnemann   *Rosa. W. Hobhouse*

Homoeopathy-Complete Handbook   *K.P.S.Dhama*

        and Suman Dhama

Tit Bits of Homoeopathy   *T.P.Chatterjee*

Highlights of Homoeopathic Practicing   *T.P. Chatterjee*

Snapshot Prescriber   *A.C. Dutta*

Chumbuk Chikitsa   *M.T.Santwani*

Acupressure   *Dha. Ra. Gala, D.Gala and S. Gala*

Practioner's Guide to Gall Bladder Stones and   *Shiv Dua*

Kidney Stones

Oral Diseases   *Shiv Dua*

Know and Solve Your Thyroid Problems   *Shiv Dua*

(Under publication)